Surgery for Pancreatic and Associated Carcinomata

Single Surgical Procedures 4

A Colour Atlas of

Surgery for Pancreatic and Associated Carcinomata

(Whipple's procedure and operations for neoplasms of the pancreas, lower bile duct, and ampulla of Vater)

T. Vincent Taylor

Walter de Gruyter · Berlin · New York 1984

T. Vincent Taylor MD, Ch. M, FRCS, FRCSE; Consultant Surgical Gastroenterologist, Manchester Royal Infirmary; Lecturer in Surgery, University of Manchester; Previously Hunterian Professor, Royal College of Surgeons of England and Moynihan Medallist. (Photography by University Department of Medical Illustration, Manchester Royal Infirmary)

Original Publishers: Wolfe Medical Publications Ltd., · London
Exclusive co-publishers for the Federal Republic of Germany and Austria: Walter de Gruyter & Co., Genthiner Strasse 13, D-1000 Berlin 30. 1984.

Printed by Royal Smeets Offset b.v., Weert, Netherlands

Cover design: Rudolf Hübler

General Editor, Wolfe Surgical Atlases:
William F. Walker, DSc, ChM, FRCS (Eng.), FRCS (Edin.), FRS (Edin.)

CIP-Kurztitelaufnahme der Deutschen Bibliothek

Taylor, T. Vincent:
A colour atlas of surgery for pancreatic and associated carcinomata / T. Vincent Taylor. –
Berlin; New York: de Gruyter, 1984.
(Single surgical procedures; 4)
ISBN 3-11-010013-4
ISBN 3-11-010012-6 (Subskr.-Pr.)
NE: GT

Contents

Acknowledgements

I am grateful to my senior colleague, Mr Bruce Torrance; Mr G. Rogers, Head of the Medical Illustration Department; Dr Helen Whitwell of the Department of Pathology, Manchester University; Dr J.G.B. Russell, Department of Radiology, Manchester Royal Infirmary and Mrs J. Mathias for typing the text.

Introduction

Halsted was the first to attempt surgical excision of an ampullary carcinoma in 1899, when he resected a segment of the second part of the duodenum and a portion of the pancreas. After this many attempts were made to perform limited resections of pancreatic tumours. However, it was not until 1935 that Whipple reported a successful two-stage procedure for radical en-bloc resection of the head of the pancreas and duodenum.

In March 1940 Whipple performed the first recorded one-stage removal of the head of the pancreas and duodenum, with occlusion of the pancreatic stump. Although many variations of the theme have been described, radical pancreatico-duodenectomy, attributed to Whipple, remains the standard operation for resectable growths of the head of the pancreas, lower end of the bile duct, and ampulla of Vater. This procedure is described herein.

This operation is curative for a high proportion of patients with carcinoma of the ampulla of Vater or the lower end of the common bile duct. It is occasionally successful, in the long-term, for early carcinomas of the pancreas but only when the tumour is well circumscribed without invasion or encapsulation of the superior mesenteric or portal veins, or lymphatic spread.

Tumours of the body and tail of the pancreas carry an even worse prognosis, as extra-glandular involvement is almost invariably present by the time the diagnosis has been made.

In recent years there has been a tendency in some centres to perform total pancreatectomy rather than Whipple's procedure. This is a more radical cancer operation and obviates the need for a pancreatic anastomosis with its attendant problems. It occasionally gives rise, however, to an unstable form of diabetes. The results have not been shown to be any better than those associated with Whipple's procedure, and most surgeons have reverted to the latter.

Percutaneous transhepatic cholangiogram (left) showing dilated intra-hepatic and common hepatic ducts. Some contrast has flowed into the dilated gallbladder. Endoscopic retrograde cholangiopancreatography (right), in the same patient, shows the extent of the partially obstructing common bile-duct tumour.

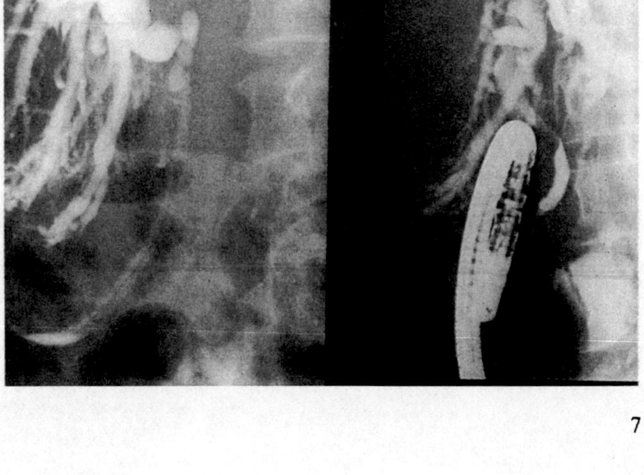

Preoperative investigations

Haematological and biochemical

Full blood count, erythrocyte sedimentation rate, urea, electrolytes, bilirubin, transaminases, alkaline phosphatase and amylase should be measured. Estimation of the patient's prothrombin time and investigation of the ability to clot are essential and these should be corrected where abnormal.

Radiological investigations

1 Plain abdominal xray and chest xray.
2 Ultrasound of the liver, biliary tract and pancreas.
3 Percutaneous transhepatic cholangiography (PTC).
4 Barium meal.
5 Endoscopic retrograde cholangio-pancreatography (ERCP).
6 Computerised tomography.
7 Selective arteriography – with views of the venous phase.

Chest xray will rule out pulmonary metastases. Ultrasound examination often reveals a tumour in the head of the pancreas with a dilated biliary tree and liver metastases may be apparent. Percutaneous transhepatic cholangiography confirms the presence of dilated bile ducts and identifies the site, nature and often extent of the stricture at the lower end of the bile duct. Widening of the duodenal loop may be seen on a barium meal, with a reversed letter '3' sign along the second part of the duodenum. An ampullary tumour may be visualised and biopsied at ERCP, and the length of the stricture may be more accurately determined when this investigation is used as an adjunct to PTC. Specimens for cytological examination may also be obtained. Computerised tomography may be a useful adjunct to ultrasound in differentiating solid from cystic lesions in the pancreas; imaging may be enhanced by using contrast media. Where doubt exists regarding the nature of a lesion in the region of the pancreatic head, selective arteriography may be valuable in demonstrating vascular encasement or displacement. This investigation is most valuable in that the venous phase demonstrates the superior mesenteric and portal veins, invasion of which by tumour is likely to preclude surgical resection. Ultrasound and computerised tomography may also be helpful in demonstrating the patency of the portal vein.

Preoperative preparation

Vitamin K

Where the patient is jaundiced, preoperative Vitamin K should be administered for several days.

Prophylactic antibiotics

Infective complications are a major cause of morbidity and mortality after such major operations. A broad-spectrum antibiotic such as cefamandole, mezlocillin or cefoxitin should be given, either intravenously or preincisionally (i.e. infiltrated along the intended site of the incision immediately after induction of anaesthesia).

Nutrition

Where weight loss has been marked and anorexia is a major feature dietary supplementation either enteral, possibly by fine bore nasogastric tube; or even parenteral nutrition, where the latter is not tolerated, should be given.

Colonic preparation

The large bowel should be cleared by purgation or an enema.

Anaemia

Where anaemia is marked, preoperative blood transfusion is necessary.

Complications

Pancreatic fistula This major complication has an incidence of approximately 15 per cent; it is less likely to occur where there has been total obstruction of the pancreatic duct with marked dilatation. The fistula usually discharges pure pancreatic juice along one of the drainage tracks. A catheter should be inserted into the fistulous tract and low-pressure continuous suction is applied.

Haemorrhage This may be reactionary or secondary. Reactionary haemorrhage usually occurring within 24 hours of operation may take place at the site of the gastric, pancreatic or biliary anastomosis. Haemorrhage may occur from the region of the superior mesenteric or portal vein; it occasionally results from generalised oozing in a jaundiced patient who has received a large amount of transfused blood.

Secondary haemorrhage may occur between one and three weeks of the operation; it is related to sepsis, usually around a leaking pancreatic anastomosis. Stress ulceration is a cause of gastrointestinal tract bleeding in the recovery phase. The patient's prothrombin time and platelet count should always be checked when bleeding occurs.

Biliary fistula Leakage of bile-stained fluid may occur; it usually settles spontaneously but may cause subphrenic abscess formation or occasionally lead to septicaemia.

Wound infection This complication can be reduced by the use of prophylactic antibiotics.

Diabetes A complication occurring in no more than 10 per cent of cases; the condition is usually mild.

Stomal ulceration This complication occurs in about 3 per cent of subjects. Prophylaxis against the problem has induced some surgeons to perform 70 per cent gastrectomy and others vagotomy. Indeed highly selective vagotomy with pylorus preservation has been advised.

Whipple's procedure

1

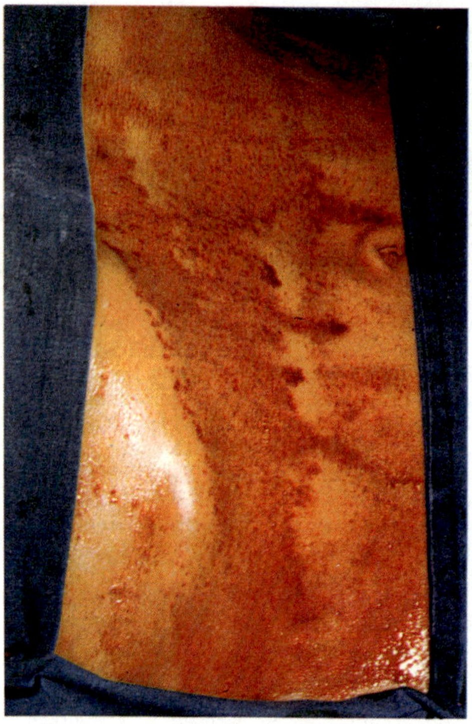

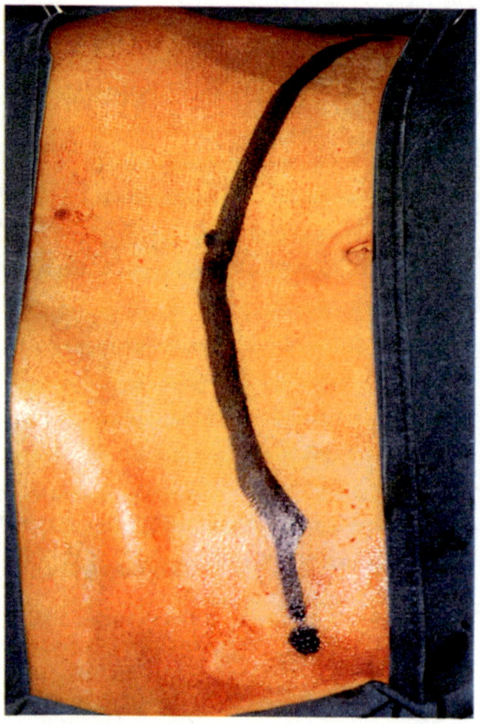

2

1 Preparation of abdomen. The abdomen is prepared with povidone iodine from one inch above the nipples down to the pubic tubercle. Drapes are applied to expose the upper abdomen from the lower end of the xiphoid process to the inferior aspect of the umbilicus, and laterally as far as the anterior axillary lines.

2 A choice of incision lies between: a transverse upper abdominal, with the possibility of a vertical midline superior extension; a right paramedian incision; or a long midline. The photographs which follow are taken from two patients undergoing the procedure; one through a transverse, the other through a right paramedian incision. The transverse upper abdominal incision will be shown in detail. This extends bilaterally and symmetrically from a midpoint situated equidistant from the lower end of the xiphoid process and the umbilicus. It is gently curved inferiorly to extend to the level of the upper aspect of the umbilicus, just medial to the anterior axillary lines.

3

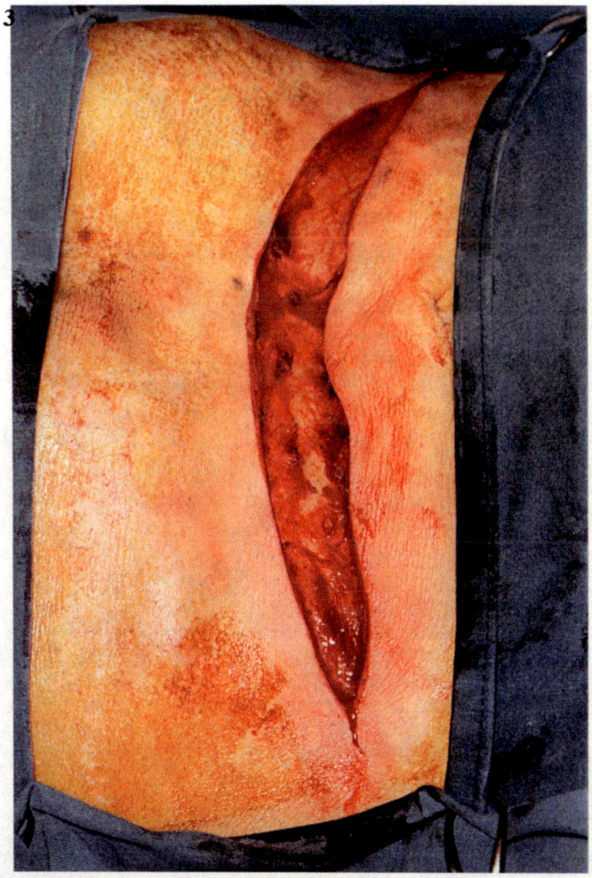

4

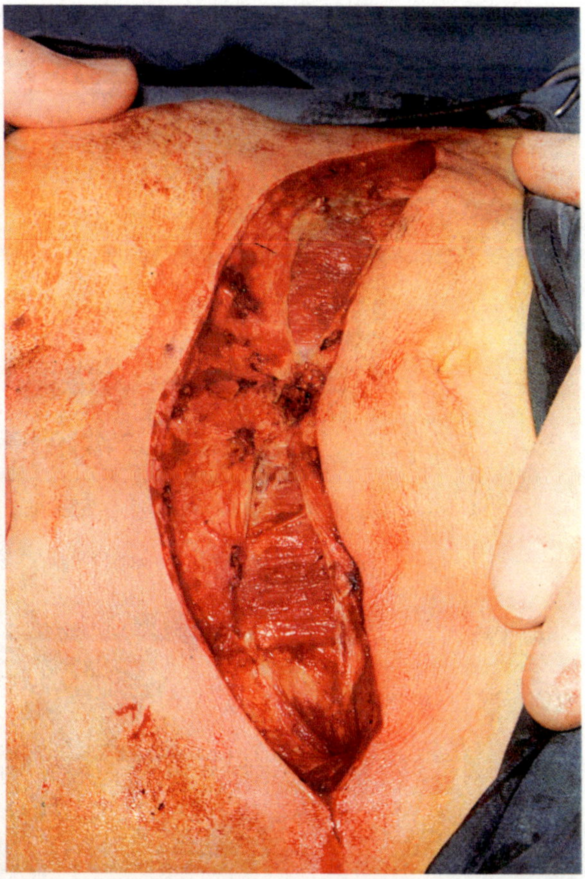

3 Skin incision. The skin superficial and deep fascia, with their intervening fatty layers, are incised to expose the anterior rectus sheath. Numerous divided small vessels are occluded with diathermy.

4 The anterior rectus sheaths are divided using diathermy to expose the rectus abdominus muscle bilaterally.

5

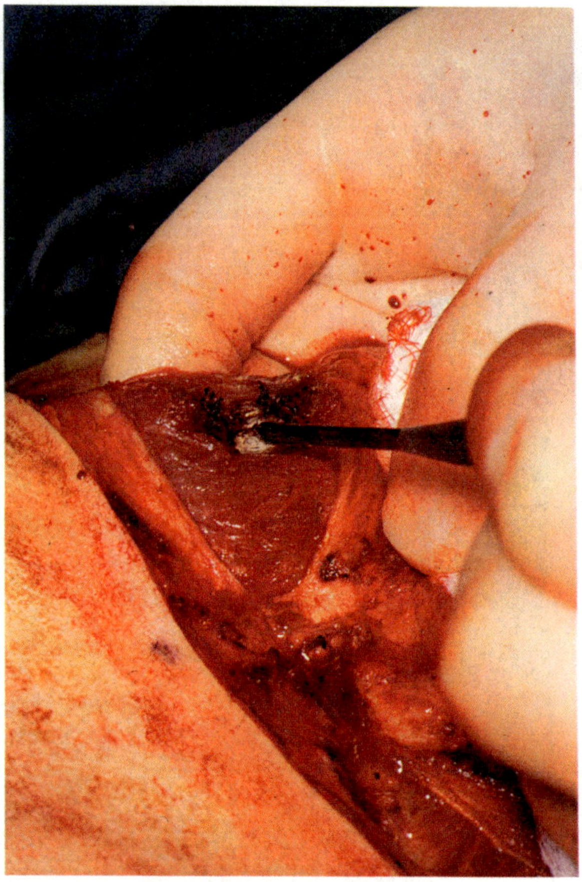

6

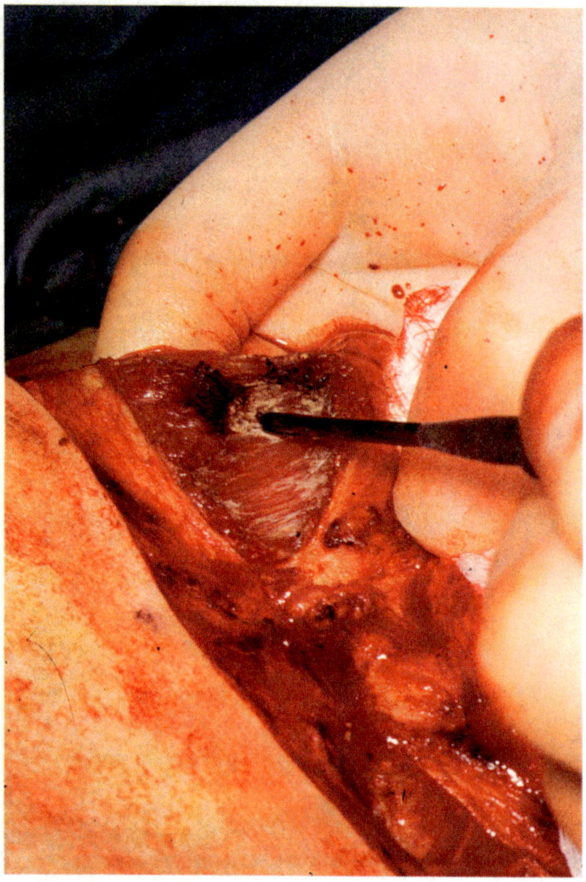

5 The anterior aspect of the rectus abdominus muscle is incised using diathermy, and the superior epigastric artery is divided and occluded.

6 Incision deepened. The incision through the muscle is gently deepened.

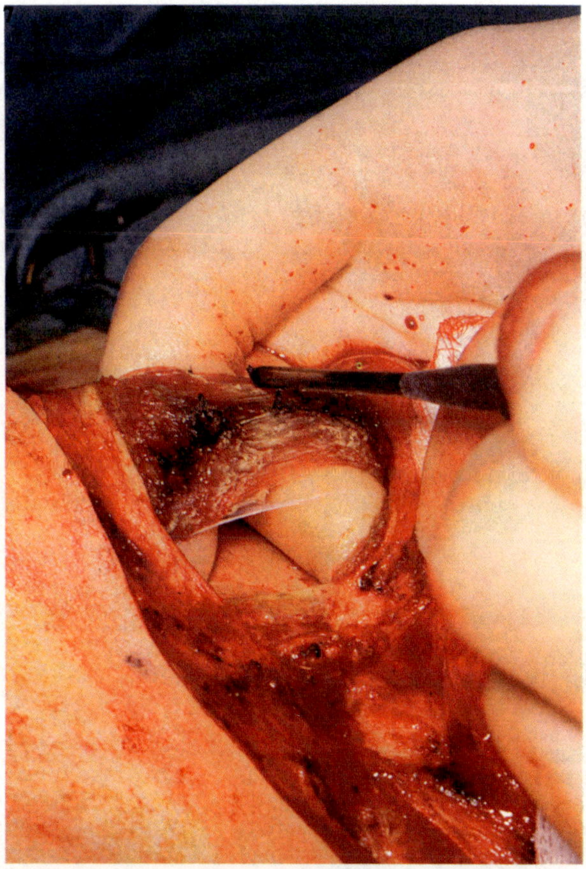

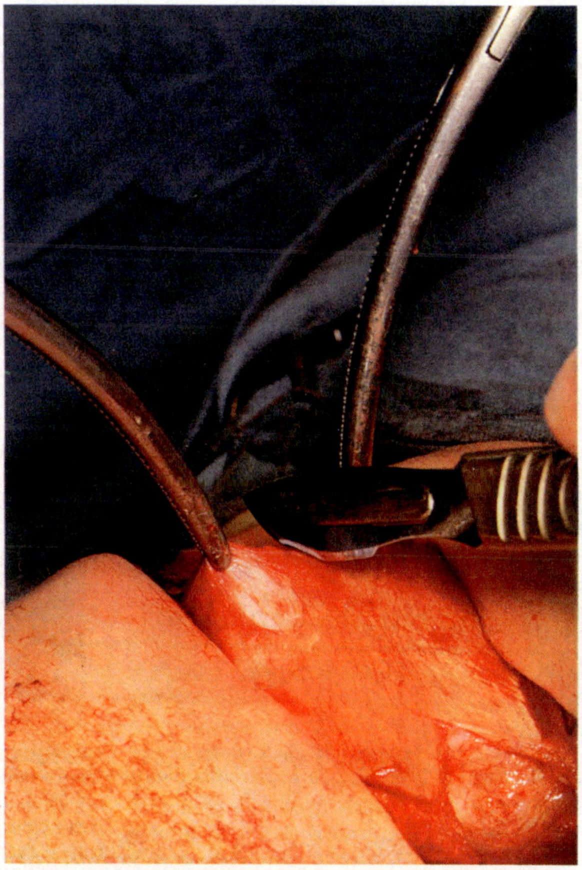

8

7 Completion of the muscular division is facilitated by anterior displacement of the rectus abdominus off the posterior rectus sheath.

8 The posterior rectus sheath is incised between artery forceps.

9

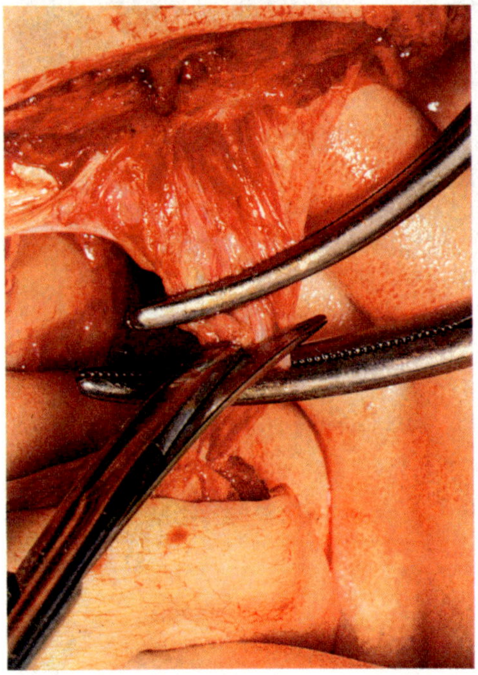

1

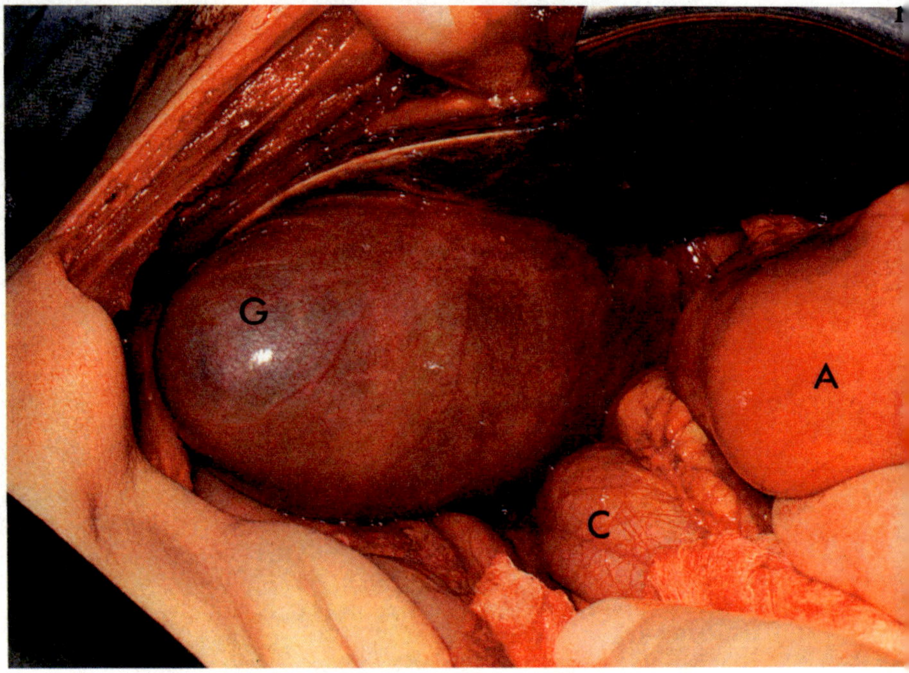

9 The falciform ligament is divided between artery forceps and ligatures are placed around these.

10 On opening the peritoneal cavity a general laparotomy is performed. The gallbladder (G) is markedly distended, confirming the theory underlying Courvoisier's law. The gastric antrum (A) can be seen to the right and the hepatic flexure of the colon (C) in the lower left of the picture.

11

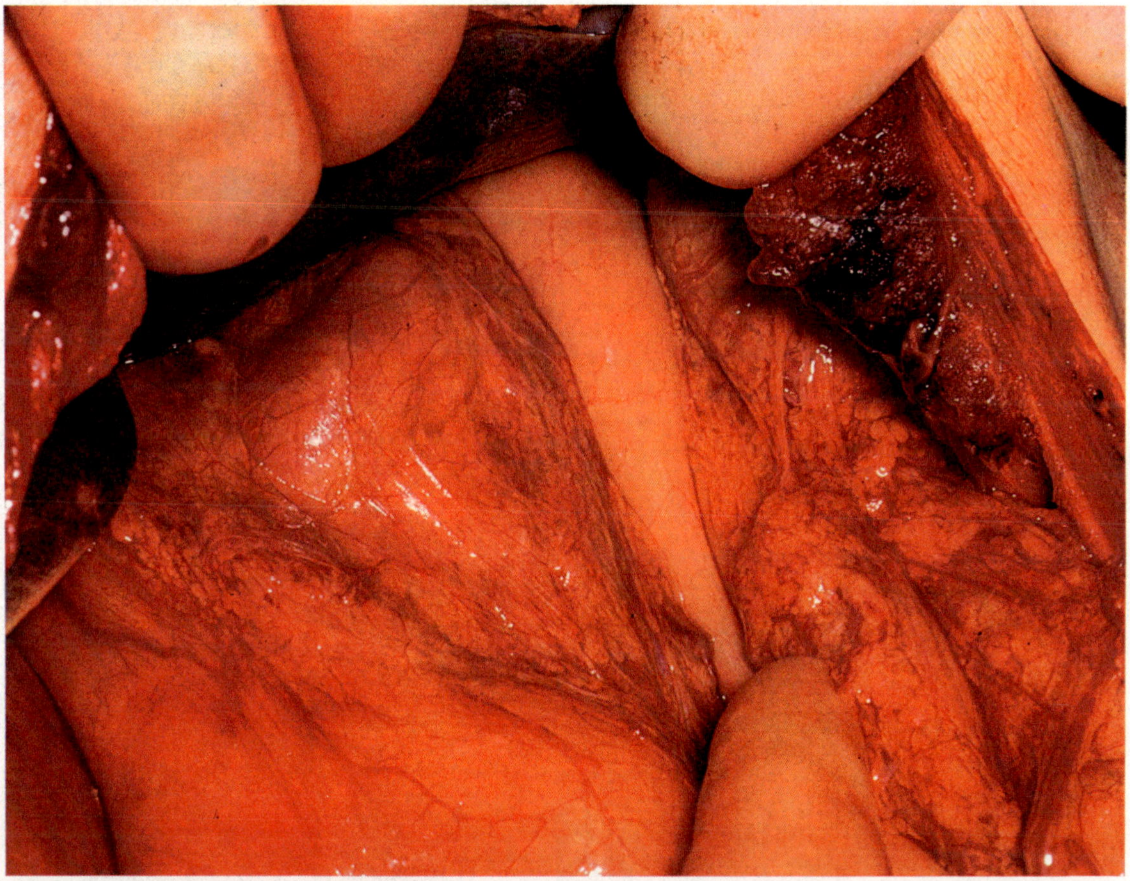

11 Through the flimsy lesser omentum the body of the pancreas can be seen, to the right of which is the lesser curvature of the stomach with branches of the nerve of Latarjet running onto it. The antrum extending across to the pylorus can be seen in the lower left of the picture. The obvious irregularity of the body of the pancreas is caused by inflammatory change in the gland and gross duct obstruction.

12 The whole operative field is seen here: a sling has been placed around the dilated common bile duct, the body of the pancreas (P) can be seen in the top right, the gastric antrum occupies the middle of the field, and the transverse mesocolon the lower part.

12

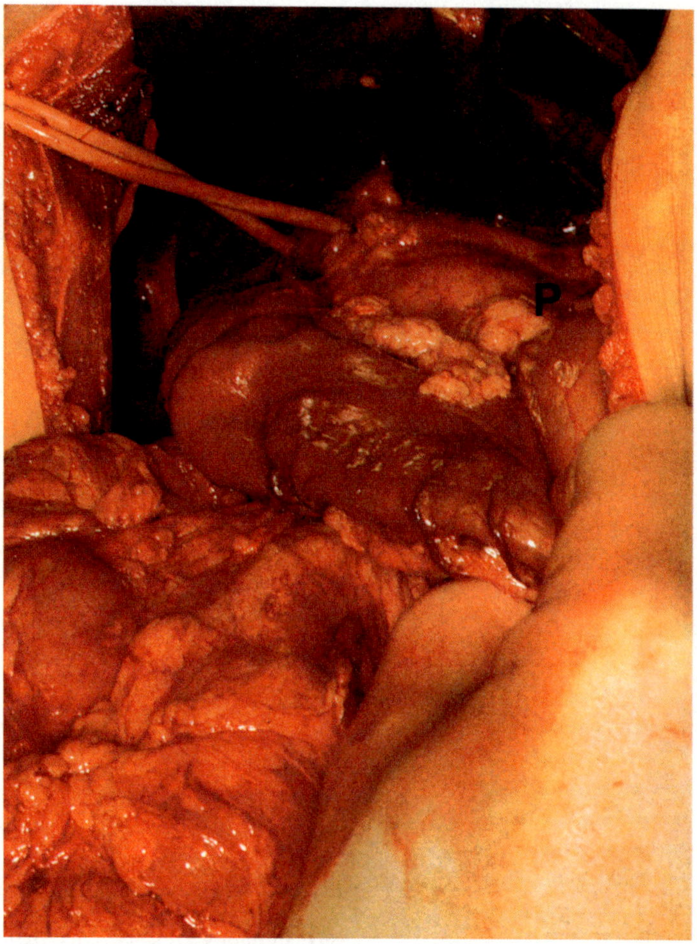

13 The transverse colon has been lifted out of the peritoneal cavity to facilitate inspection and assessment of the tumour field. This is the exposure obtained through a right paramedian incision, rather than the transverse.

13

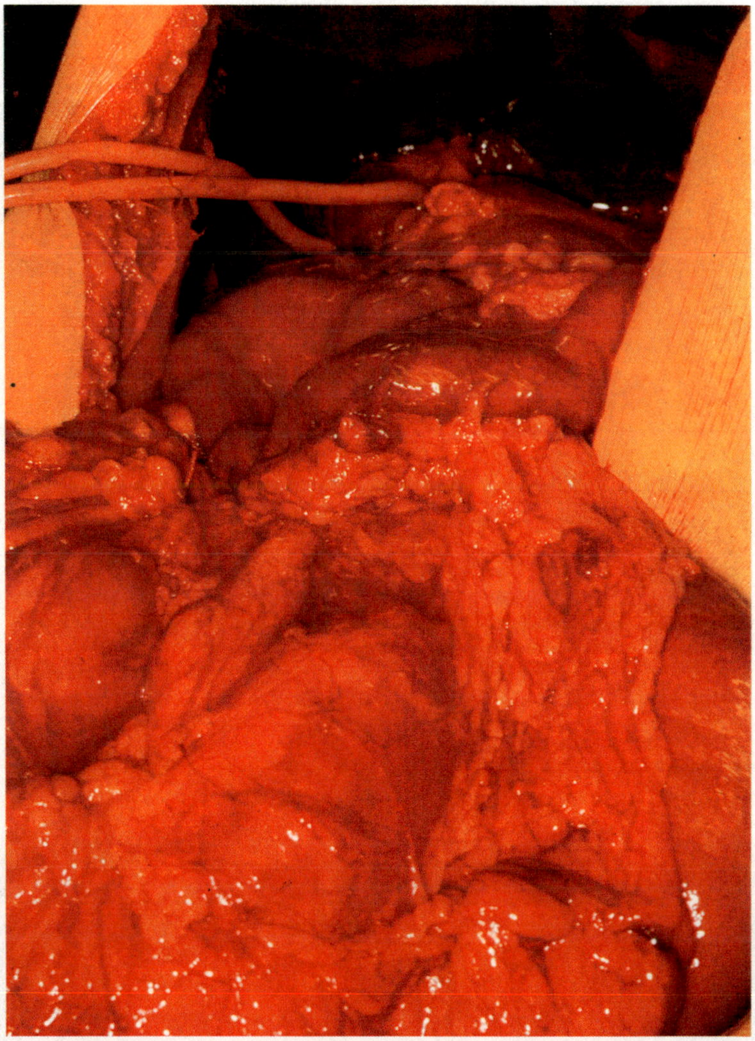

14 The hepatic flexure of the colon is retracted caudally to facilitate exposure of the second part of the duodenum.

14

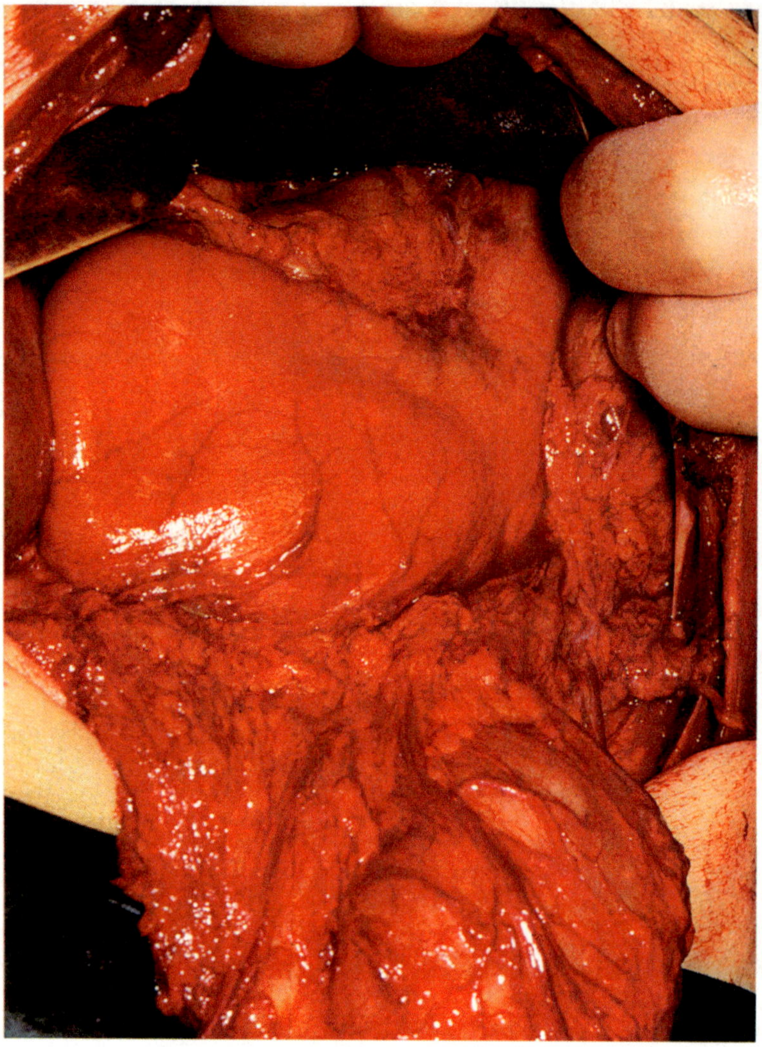

15 The anterior aspect of the tumour bearing area is carefully inspected. The site and size of the tumour in the pancreatic head is assessed; a search is made along the lesser and greater curvatures of the stomach for enlarged lymph nodes. The lesser and greater omenta are also carefully examined; a preliminary assessment is made for fixation of the tumour. Any lymph node suspected of containing tumour is excised and dispatched for frozen section.

15

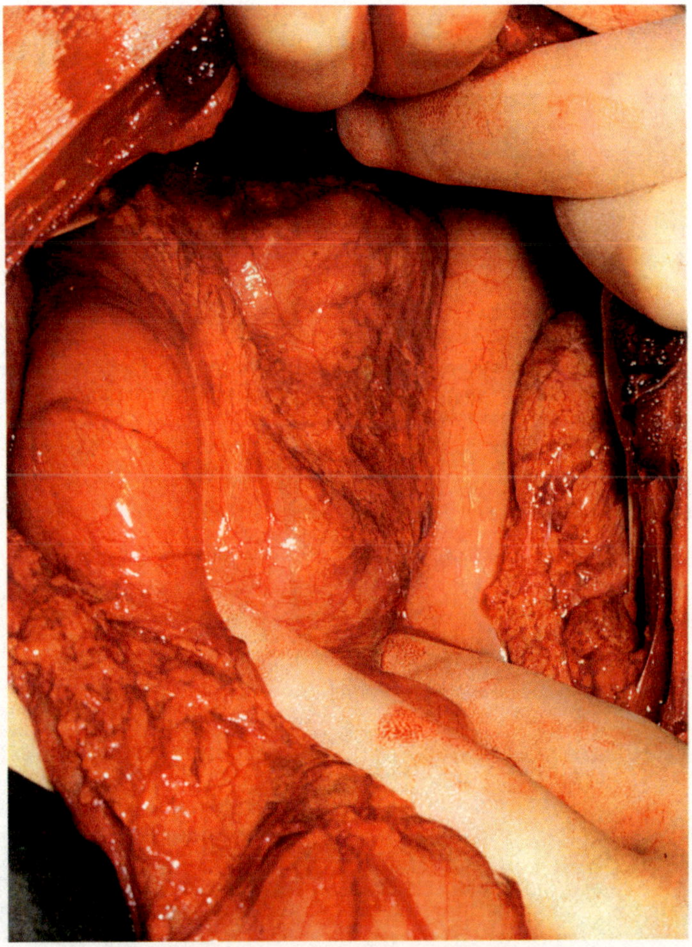

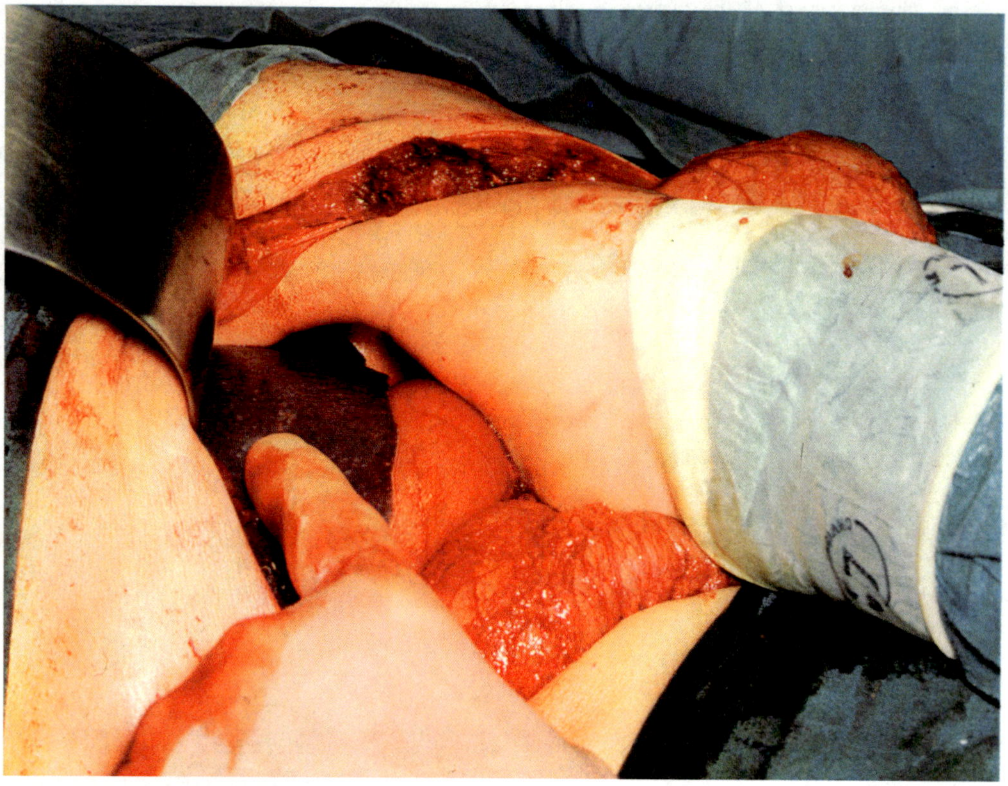

16 The liver is assessed for any evidence of metastatic deposits. When metastases have occurred to either the lymph nodes or the liver, then the operation of radical pancreatico-duodenectomy should be abandoned, and a biliary bypass is then performed to relieve jaundice.

17

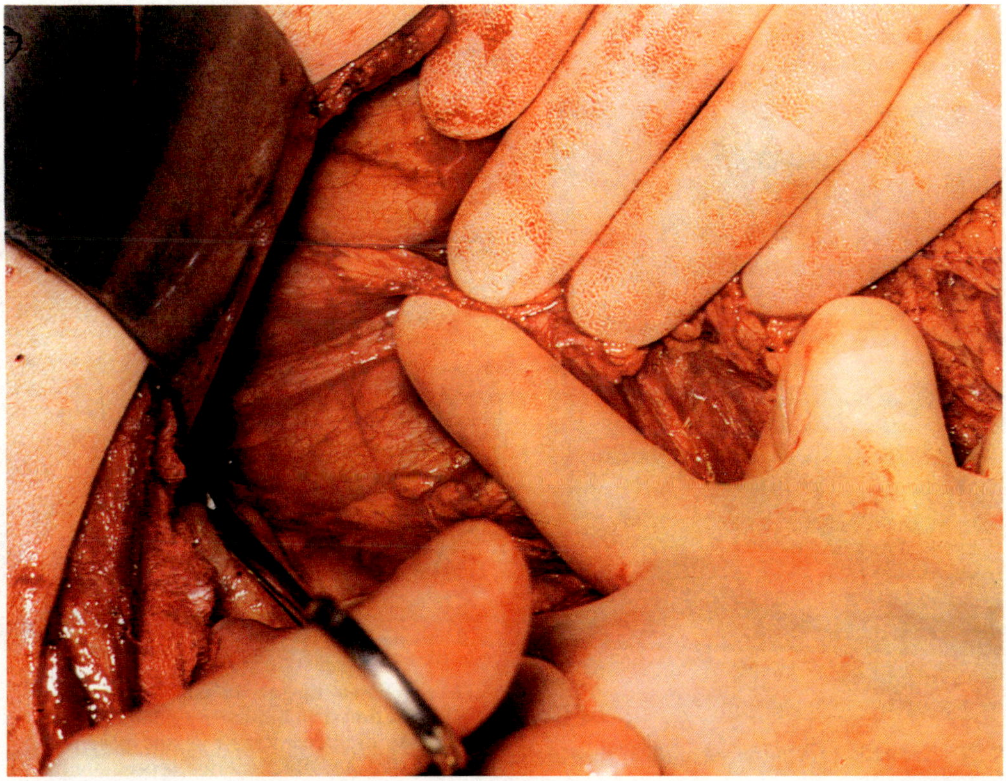

17 Mobilisation of duodenal loop and pancreatic head. The primary tumour cannot be properly assessed until the duodenal loop and head of the pancreas have been mobilised. The peritoneum, lateral to the duodenum, is incised along the length of the second part of the duodenum.

18 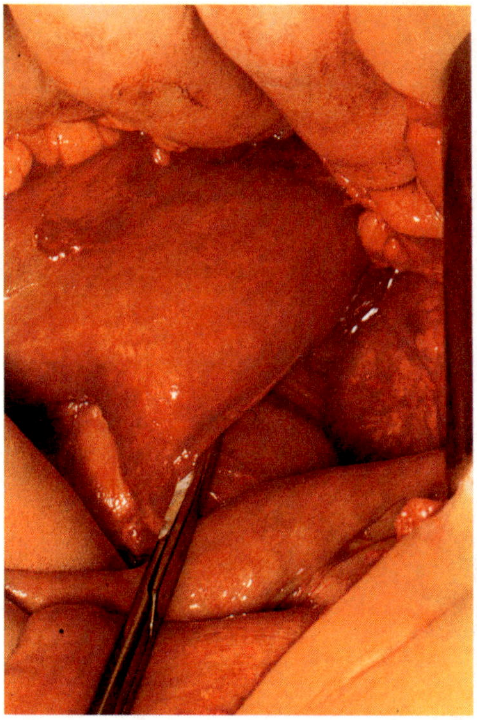

18 **The second part of the duodenum may then be lifted anteriorly.**

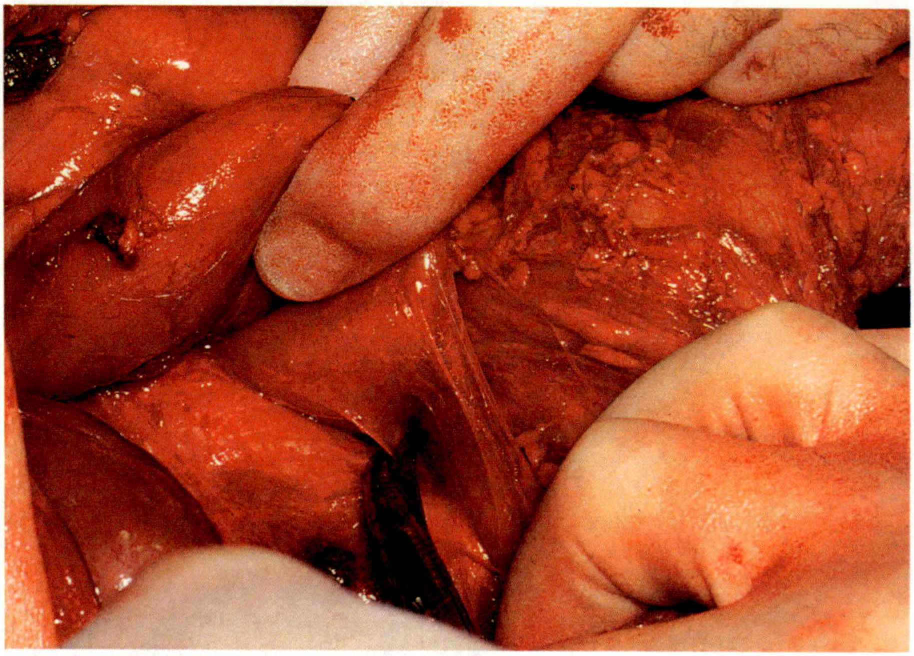

19 **The junction of the second and third parts of the duodenum is next mobilised;** avascular bands of areolar tissue are separated from the posterior abdominal wall and the anterior aspect of the inferior vena cava.

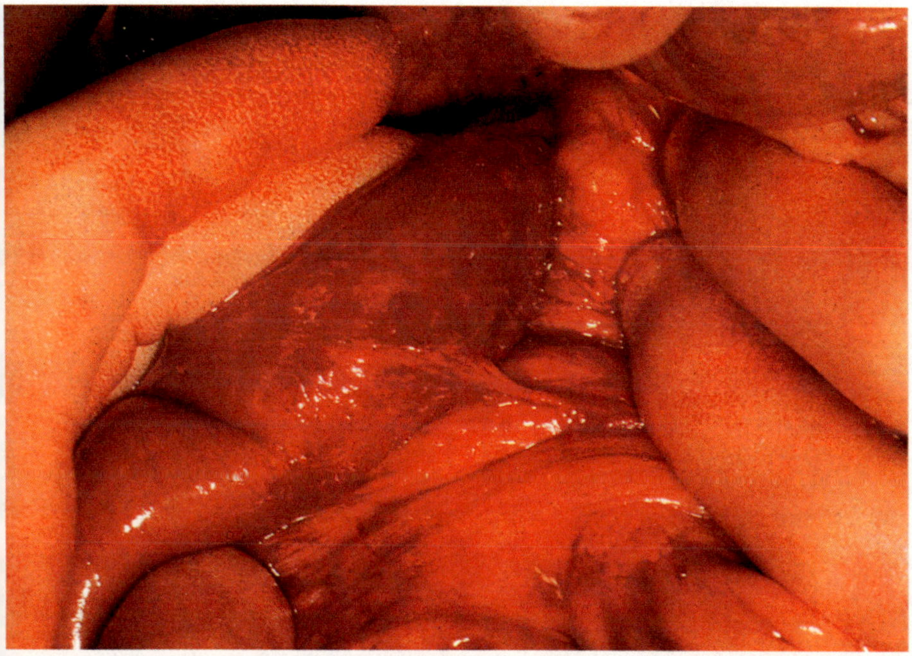

20 The mobilisation is continued by blunt dissection behind the first part of the duodenum and the pylorus.

21

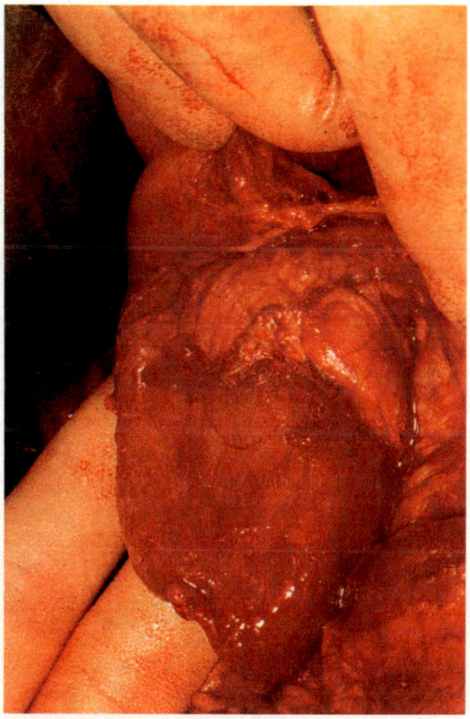

21 Further blunt dissection behind the pancreatic head allows a more detailed inspection of the size, fixation, and invasion of the tumour. The feasibility of continuing with the operation at this stage, however, remains in doubt as the crucial factor, invasion of the portal vein, cannot yet fully be assessed.

22

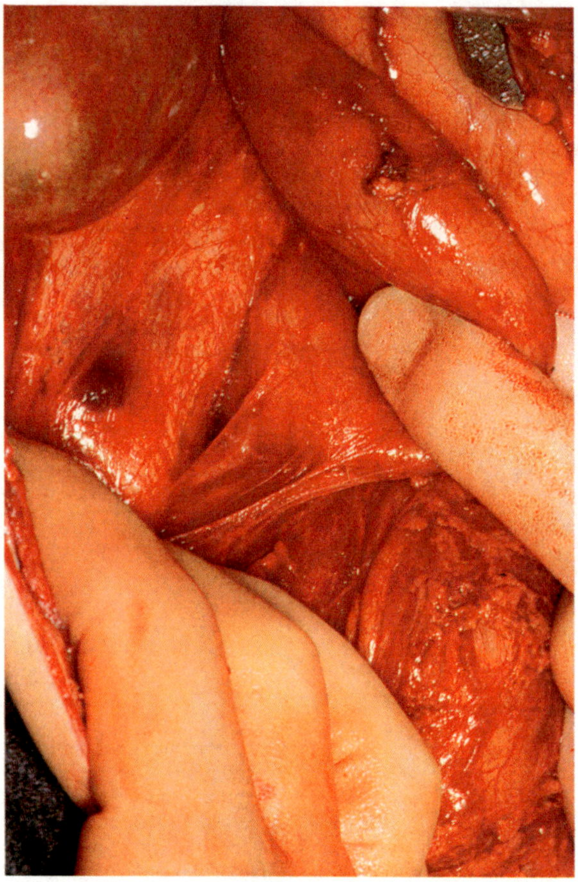

22 The duodenal loop and head of the pancreas are next mobilised as far as the midline.

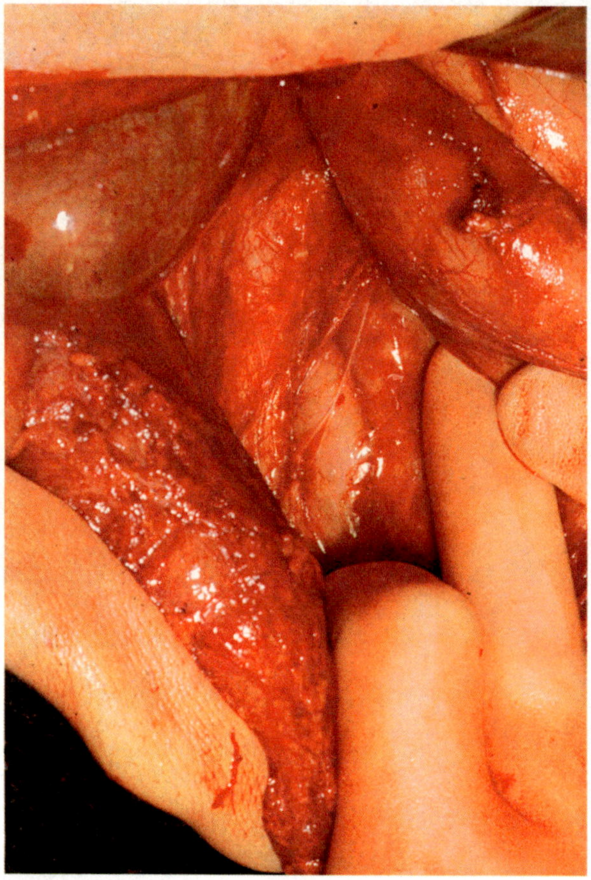

23 Further blunt dissection reveals both the inferior vena cava and the aorta. The third part of the duodenum is reflected off the anterior aspect of the aorta by blunt, finger dissection.

24

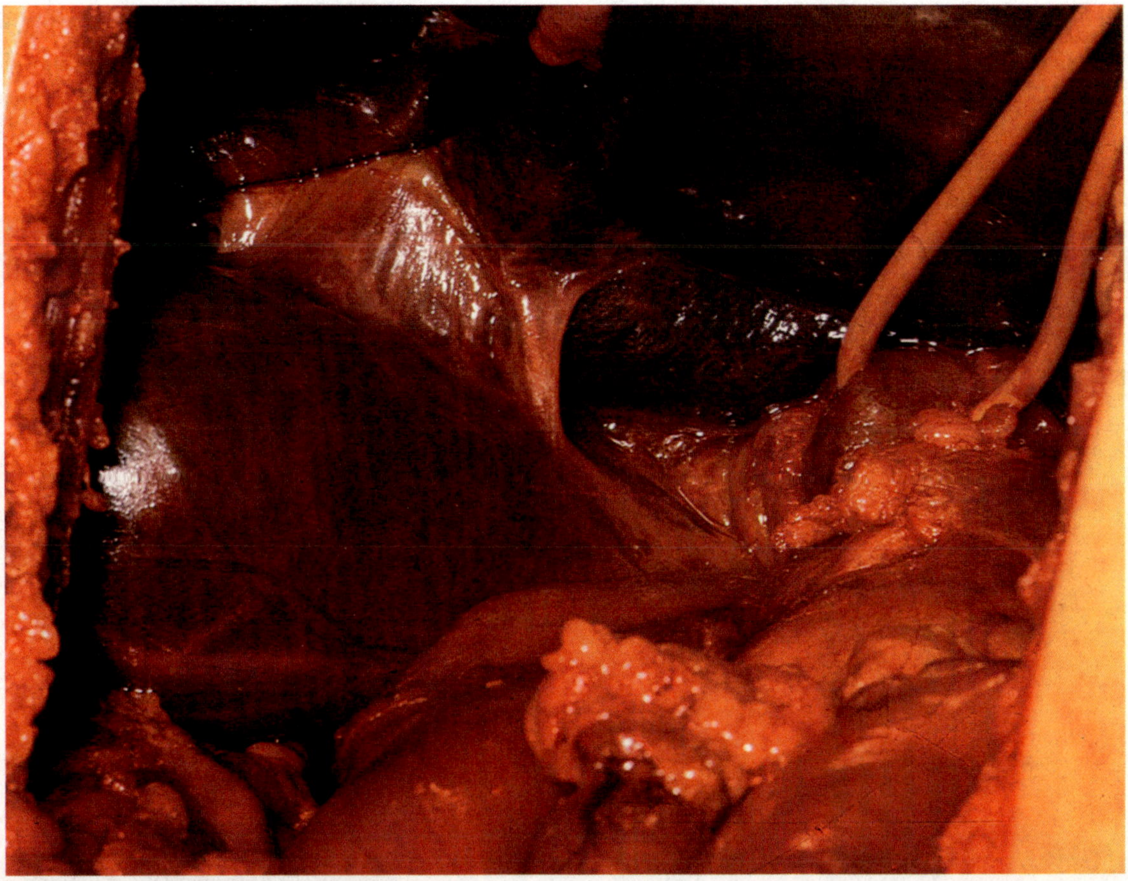

24 An assessment of the porta hepatis is next made for evidence of lymph node involvement; a sling is placed around the dilated common hepatic duct or the supraduodenal portion of the common bile duct.

25 The areolar tissue over the anterior aspect of the common bile duct is next incised and dissected free to expose the supraduodenal component of the common bile duct and the common hepatic artery which passes to the left.

25

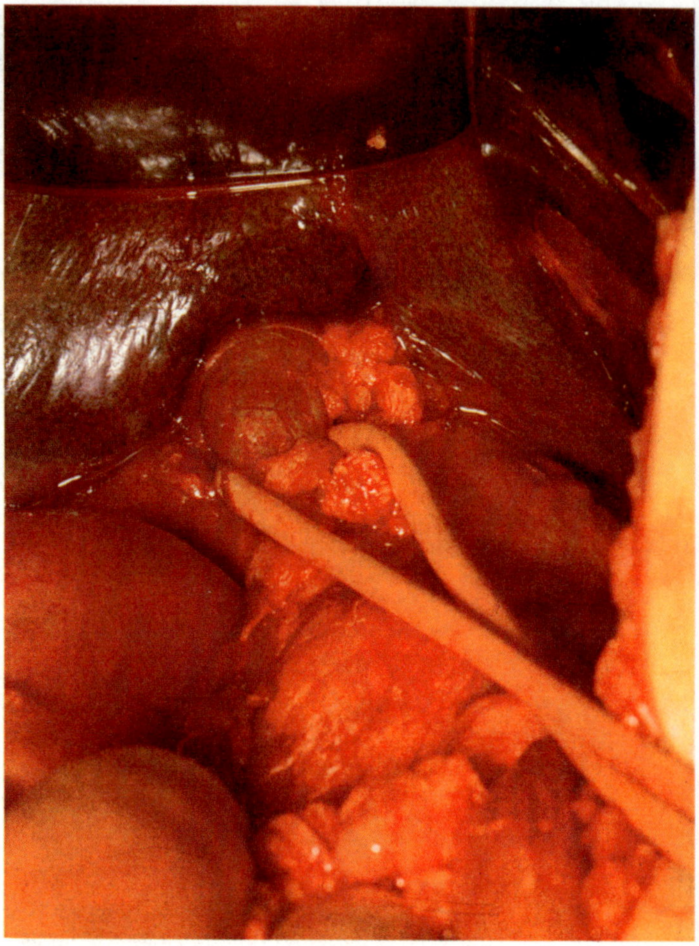

26

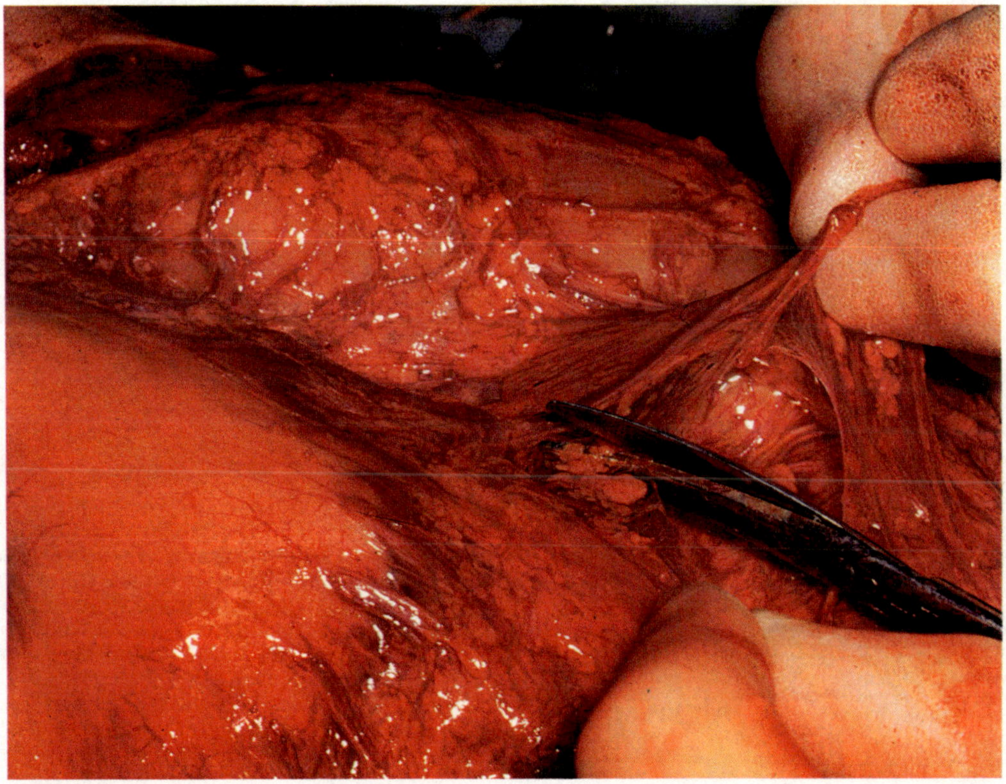

26 Mobilisation of greater curvature of stomach. If no obvious tumour spread has been found at this stage, the operation may proceed by mobilisation of the greater curvature of the stomach. An avascular area of omentum is incised outside the gastroepiploic arch, and the lesser sac of the peritoneum is opened from this aspect.

27

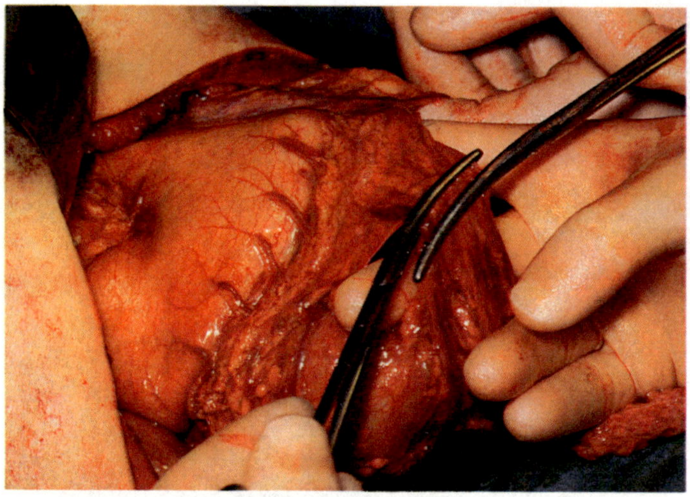

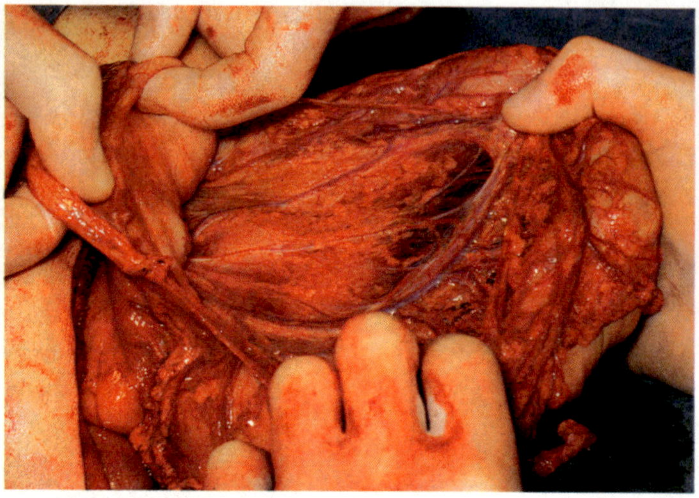

27 Vessels in the gastrocolic omentum along the lower half of the greater curvature of the stomach are next divided and ligated outside the right and left gastroepiploic vessels from the mid-body of the stomach. The stomach is then reflected forwards; avascular bands of fibrous and areolar tissue between the posterior aspect of the lesser curvature of the stomach and the anterior aspect of the body of the pancreas are incised with scissors.

28 The middle colic vessels are now exposed and along with them whitish lymphatics can be seen in the colonic mesentery. The marginal artery runs along the mesenteric aspect of the colonic mesentery. The middle colic vessels are carefully preserved; blunt dissection in the base of the mesentery reveals the superior mesenteric vessels passing anterior to the third part of the duodenum at the point of its currently most lateral mobilisation. The fourth part of the duodenum can be seen shining through the mesentery, behind and beyond the middle colic vessels.

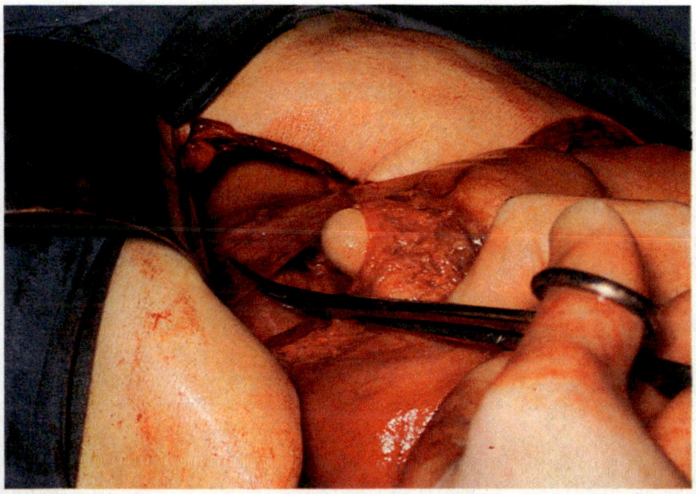

29 The avascular plane of the lesser omentum is incised between the right and left gastric arteries. This dissection is carried on to the most proximal half of the stomach. The wound at this point has been extended superiorly along the midline, to the level of the xiphisternum.

30

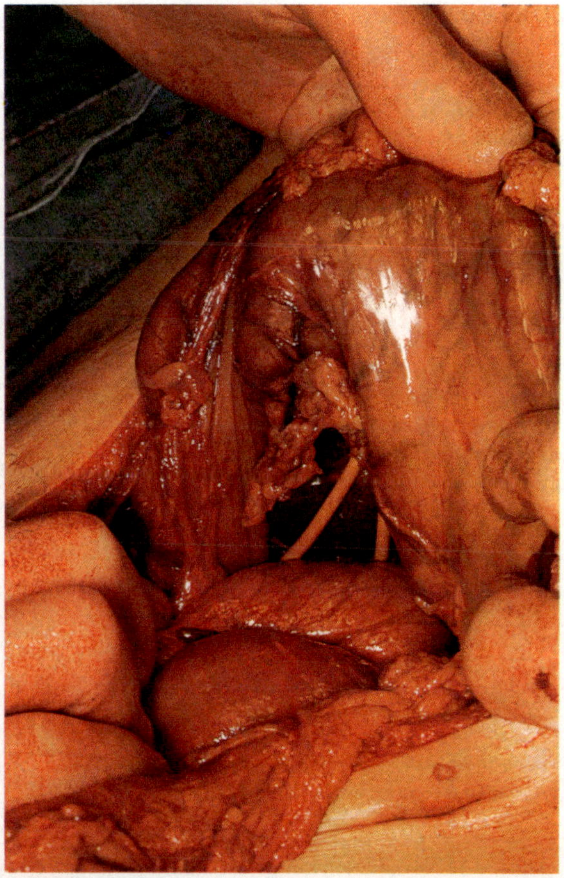

30 The right gastric artery is next ligated and divided, allowing the stomach to be reflected off the body and head of the pancreas.

31 Gastroduodenal artery clamped, divided, and ligated. Having identified the common hepatic artery and mobilised the lesser curvature of the stomach as far as the first part of the duodenum, the gastroduodenal artery is next clamped, divided, and ligated.

31

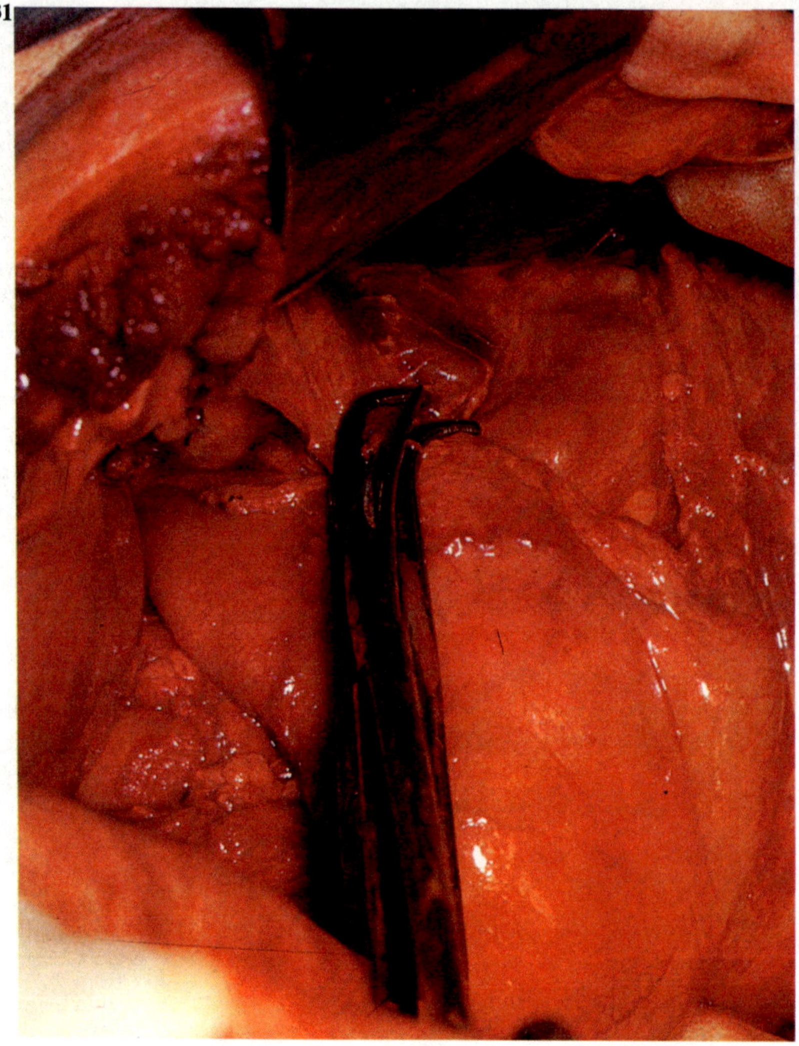

32 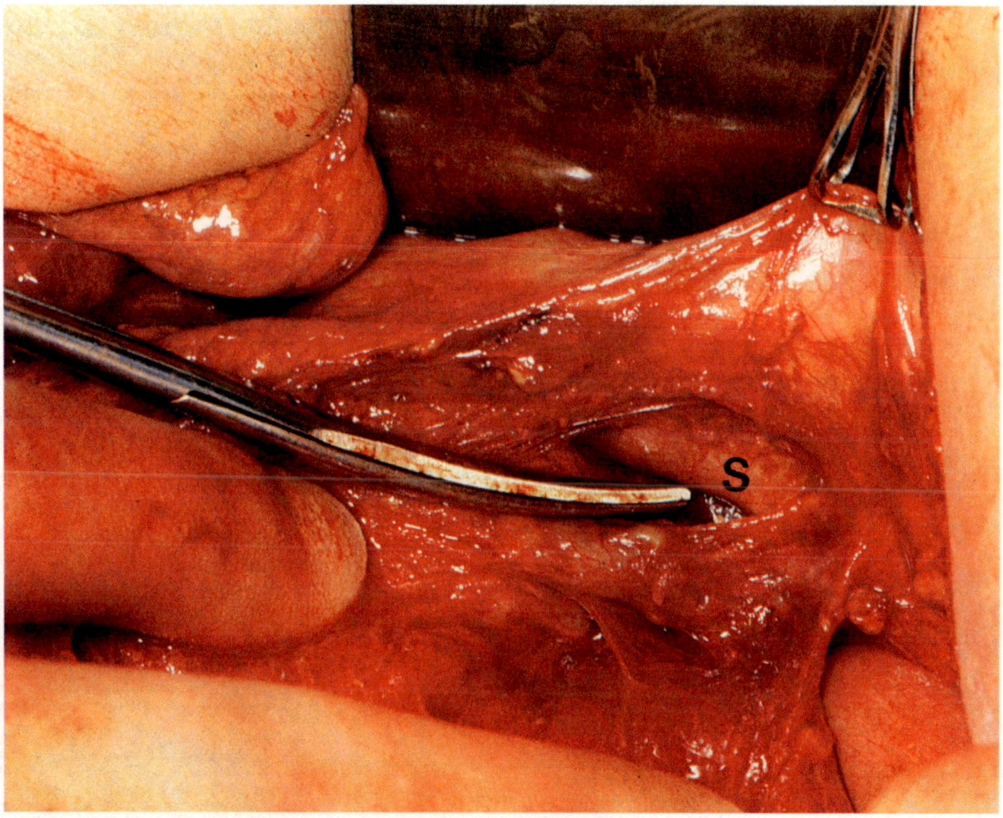

32 Attention is now turned to the mobilisation of the neck and adjacent area of the body of the pancreas. The pancreatic duct is usually markedly dilated and a variable degree of parenchymal atrophy will have occurred. The body of the pancreas is elevated just to the left of the superior mesenteric vessels; division of some avascular fibro-fatty tissue will reveal the termination of the splenic vein (S), which runs along the postero-superior aspect of the pancreas.

33

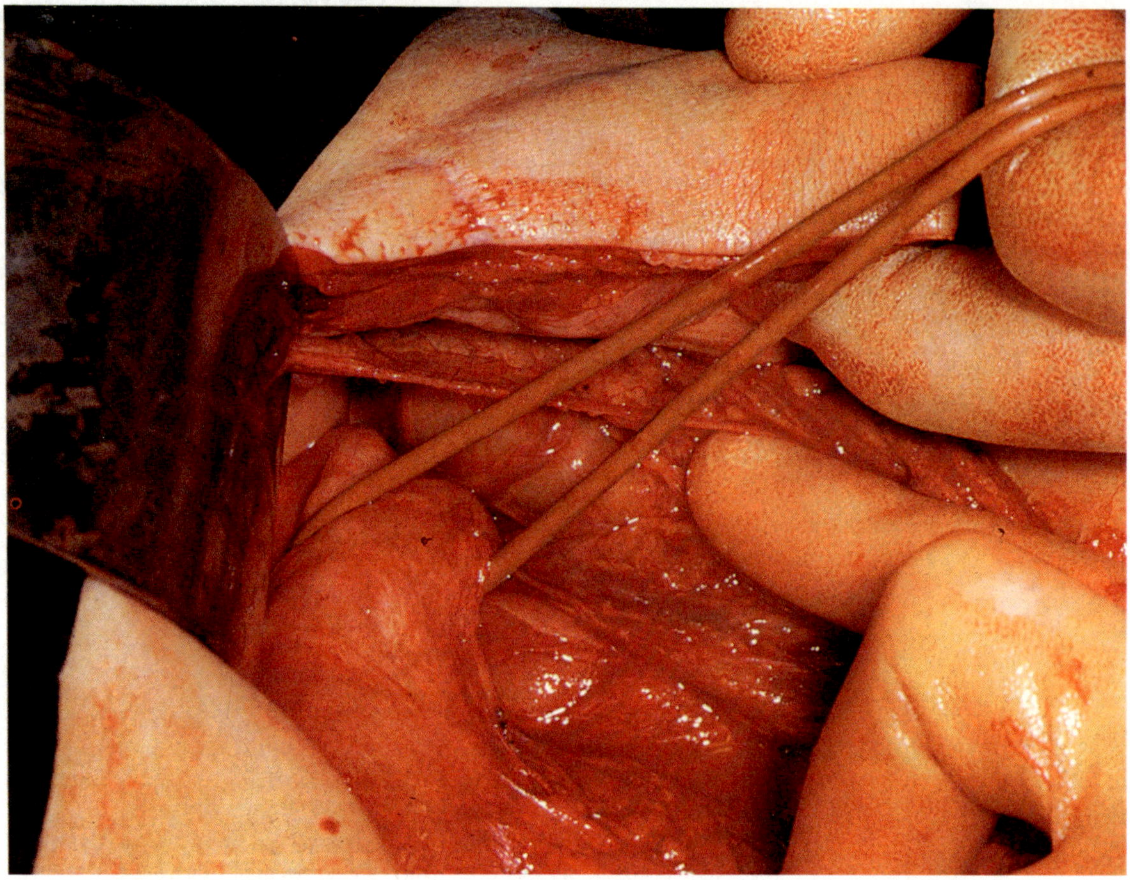

33 **Mobilisation of the neck of the pancreas** is further facilitated by blunt dissection, inserting the index finger directly behind the pancreas, and a sling being placed around the gland at this point.

The neck and body of the ncreas can be freed by blunt ssection over a distance of out 2 to 4 cm. This facili-tes both further dissection, sessment of the tumour d its relation to the portal in, and the subsequent rformance of the pancreatic astomosis.

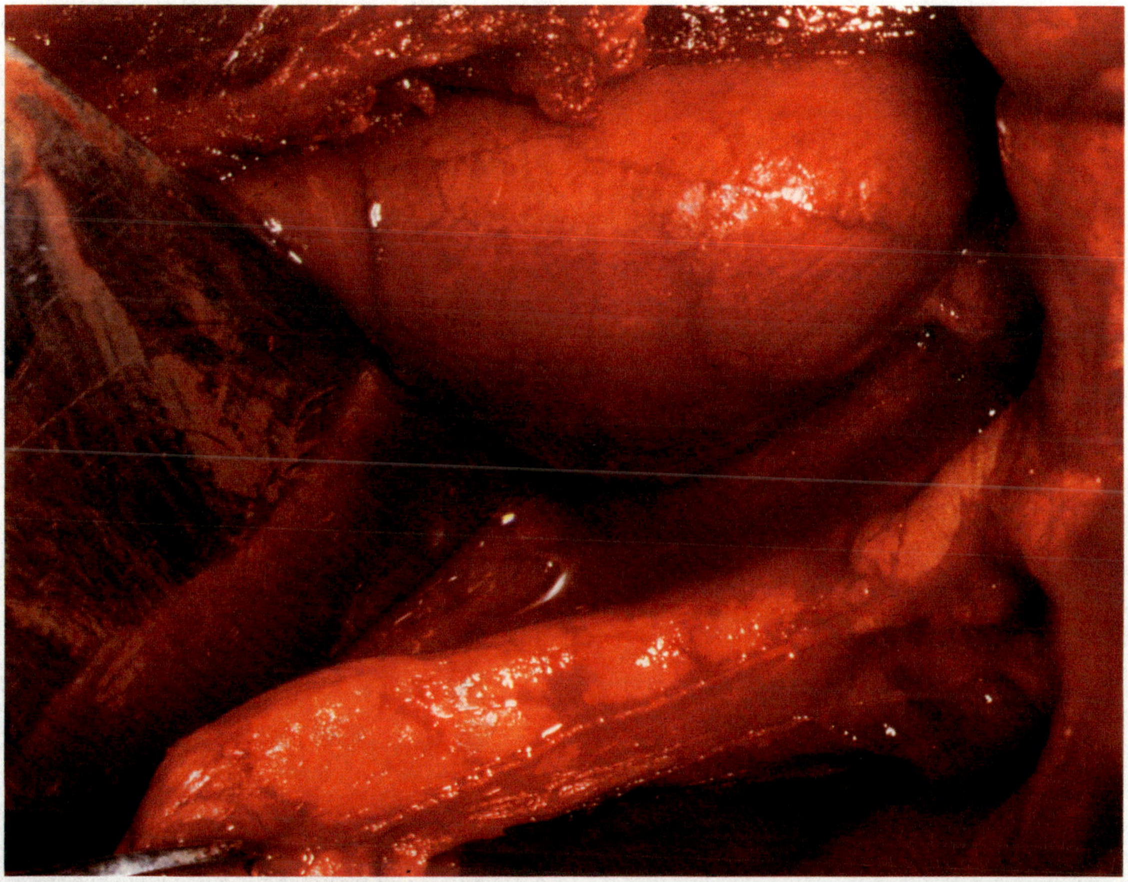

34

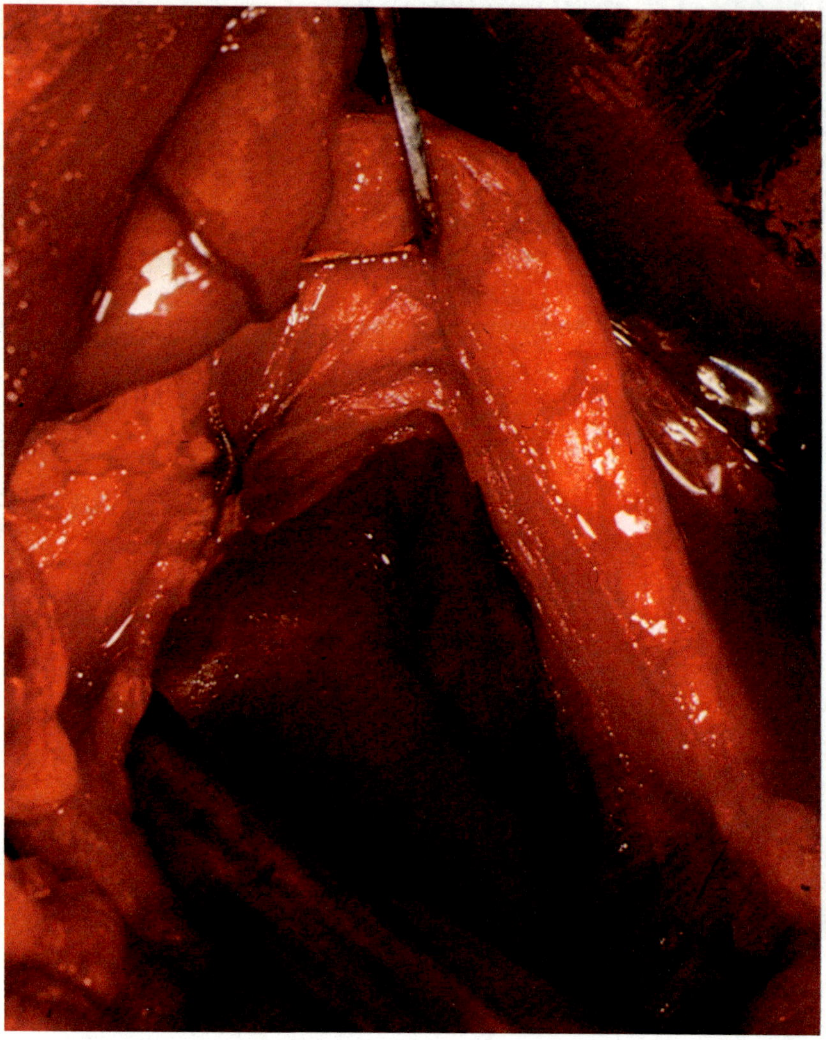

35 By lifting the pancreas forwards an excellent view is obtained of the superior mesenteric, splenic and the origin of the portal vein. A glass sucker can be seen in the left of the picture; the pancreas is elevated with Babcock's forceps. The surgeon will now be able to assess quite accurately the feasibility of mobilising the tumour from the portal vein. At this stage of the operation still no irrevocable steps have been taken; extrinsic encasement of the portal vein or superior mesenteric vessels, precluding further resection, would still allow the surgeon to perform a simple biliary diversion. The anterior aspect of the superior mesenteric and portal veins can be dissected free of the pancreas. Along the right side of the portal and superior mesenteric veins, several small veins sharply enter the pancreas; these veins require ligation after division of the pancreatic neck.

36

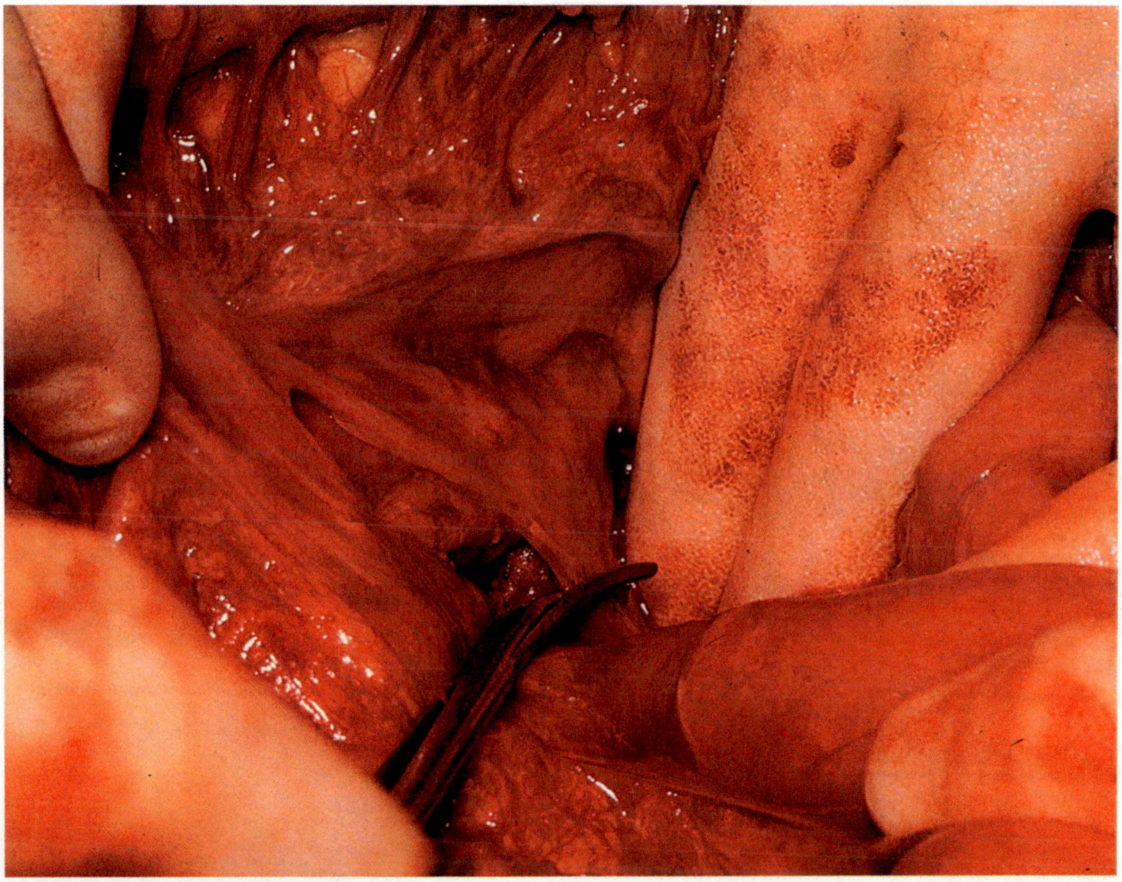

36 The distal aspect of the third part of the duodenum and the proximal jejunum are next mobilised beneath the transverse mesocolon and alongside the superior mesenteric vessels.

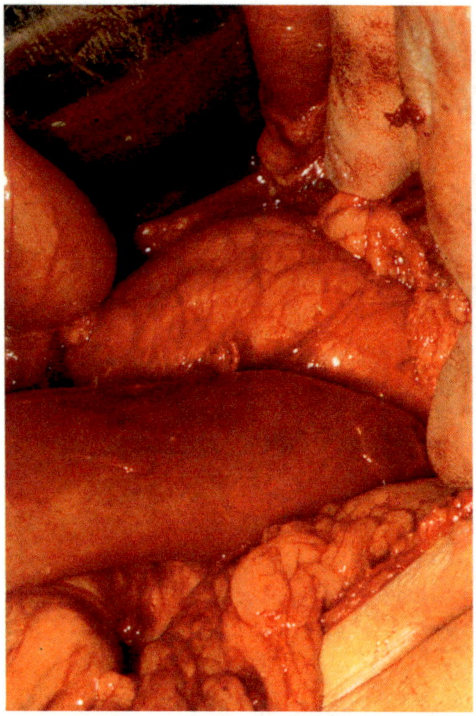

37 The dissection of the third part of the duodenum may be commenced bluntly. When the fourth part of the duodenum and proximal jejunum are encountered, vascular arcades run into these structures, as the blood supply of the gut continues from the inferior pancreaticoduodenal vessels to the proximal jejunal arcades.

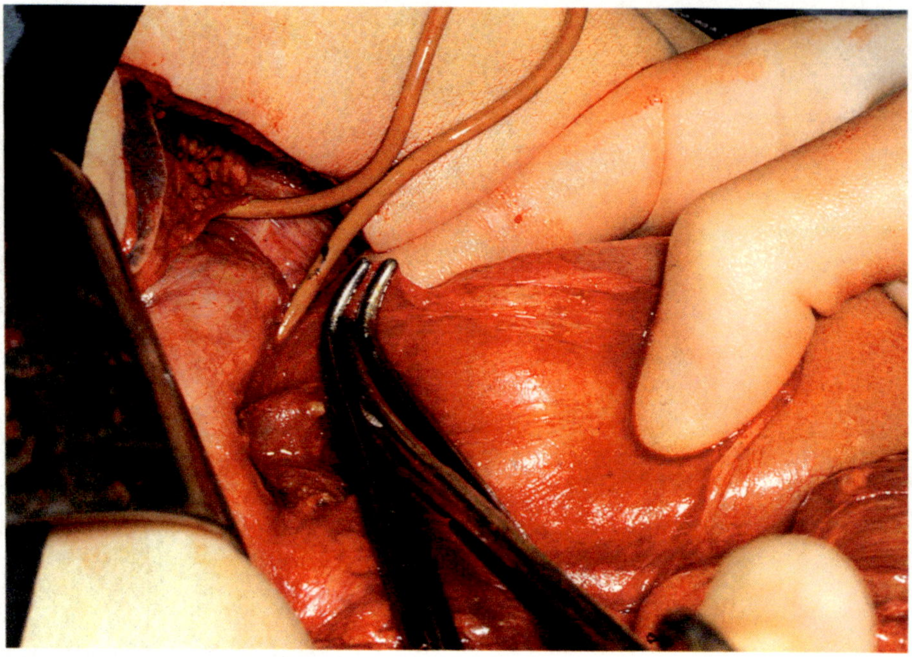

38 These vessels and the ligament of Treitz require division, which should be performed close to the bowel wall.

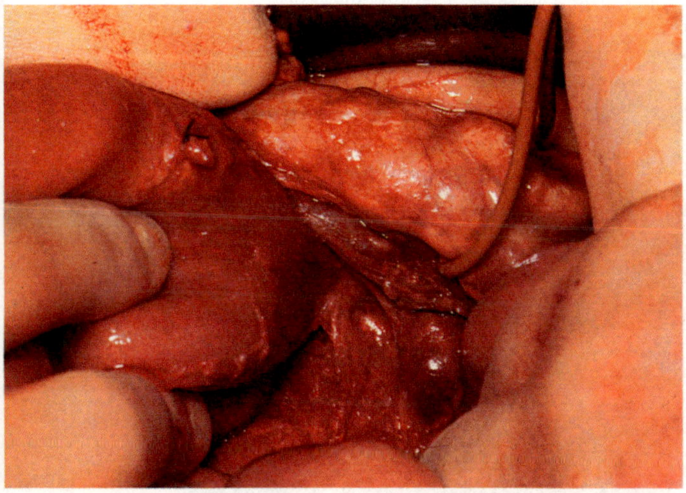

40

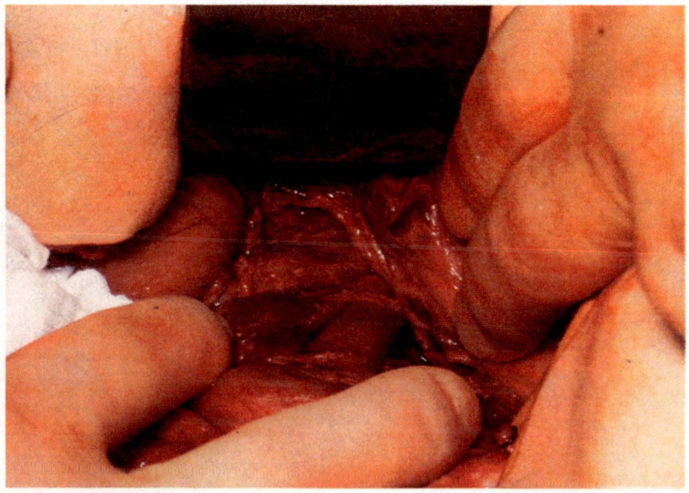

39 The mobilised bowel can be swept clear of the superior mesenteric vessels, so that the proximal jejunum is laid ready for division. This part of the dissection can be deferred until after division of the major structures, if it is felt that this is most convenient to do so.

40 The dissection is next continued along the more proximal portal vein, which is laid bare and separated from the common bile duct.

41

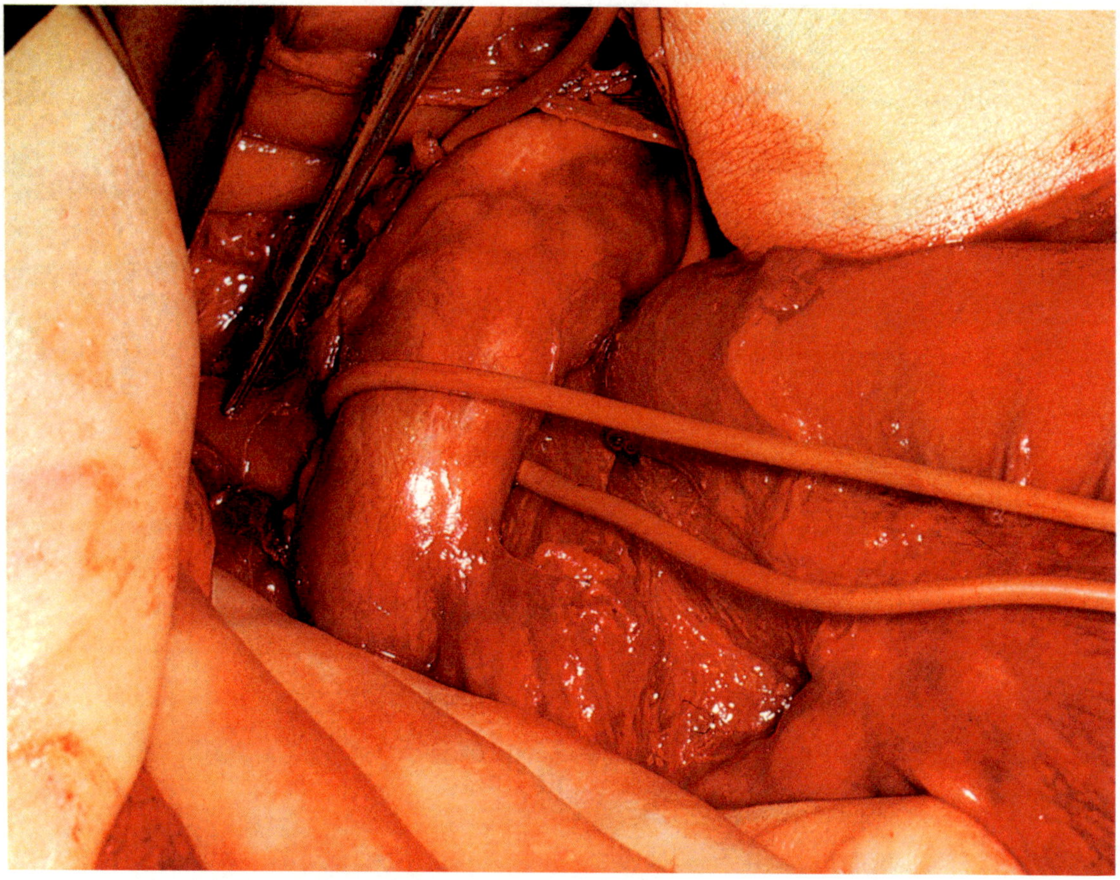

41 The neck of the pancreas is now completely separated from the surrounding structures. The posterolateral aspect of the head of the pancreas remains attached to the portal vein by a series of small veins, and the uncinate process of the gland still requires mobilisation.

42a

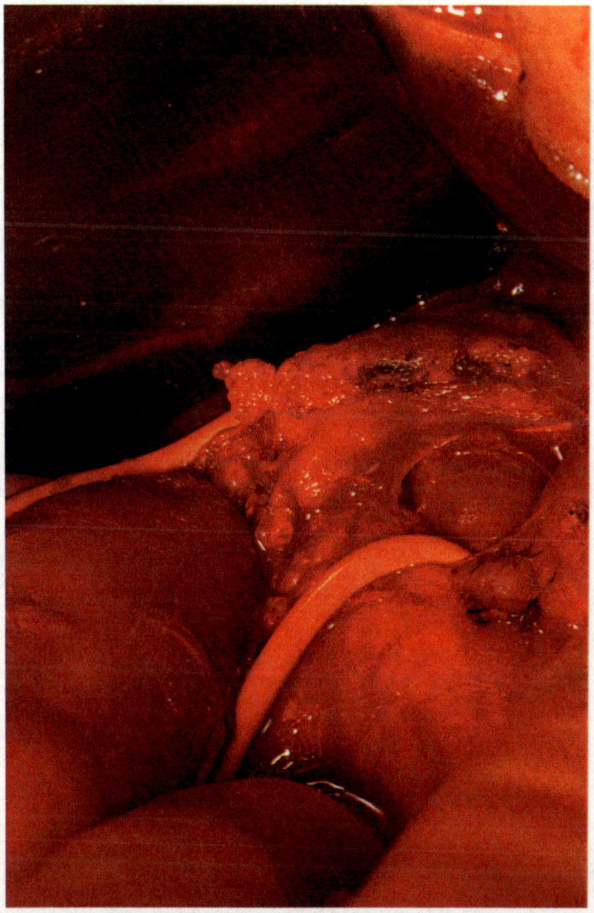

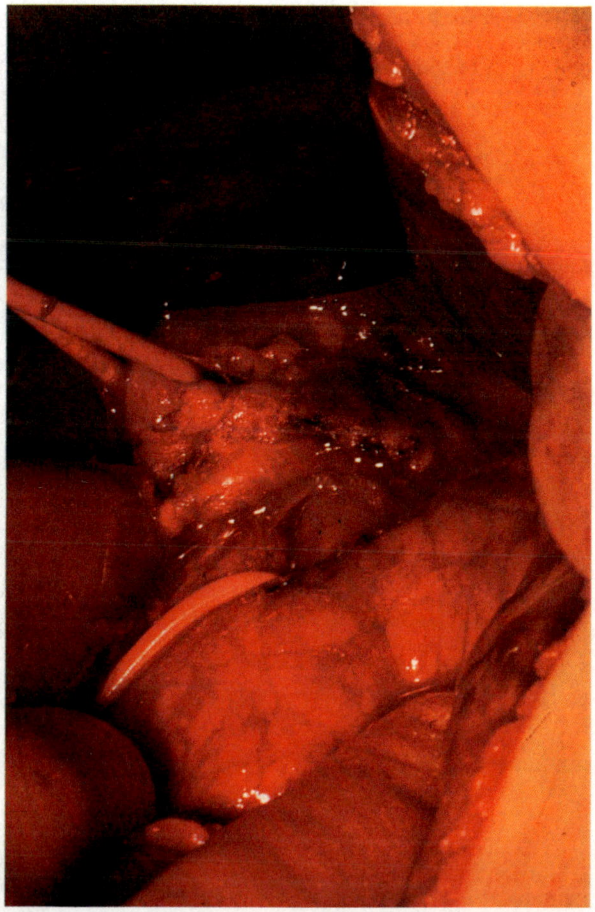

42b

42a and b Any remaining areolar and fatty tissue between the common bile duct and portal vein is divided, allowing the common hepatic artery to be displaced superomedially. The portal vein can then be freed from the posterior aspect of the common hepatic duct, up to the level of the porta hepatis, where these structures bifurcate.

43 The gallbladder is next mobilised. Before this procedure, in view of the gross dilatation of the organ, it may be considered convenient to aspirate it, using a suction trocar and cannula.

43

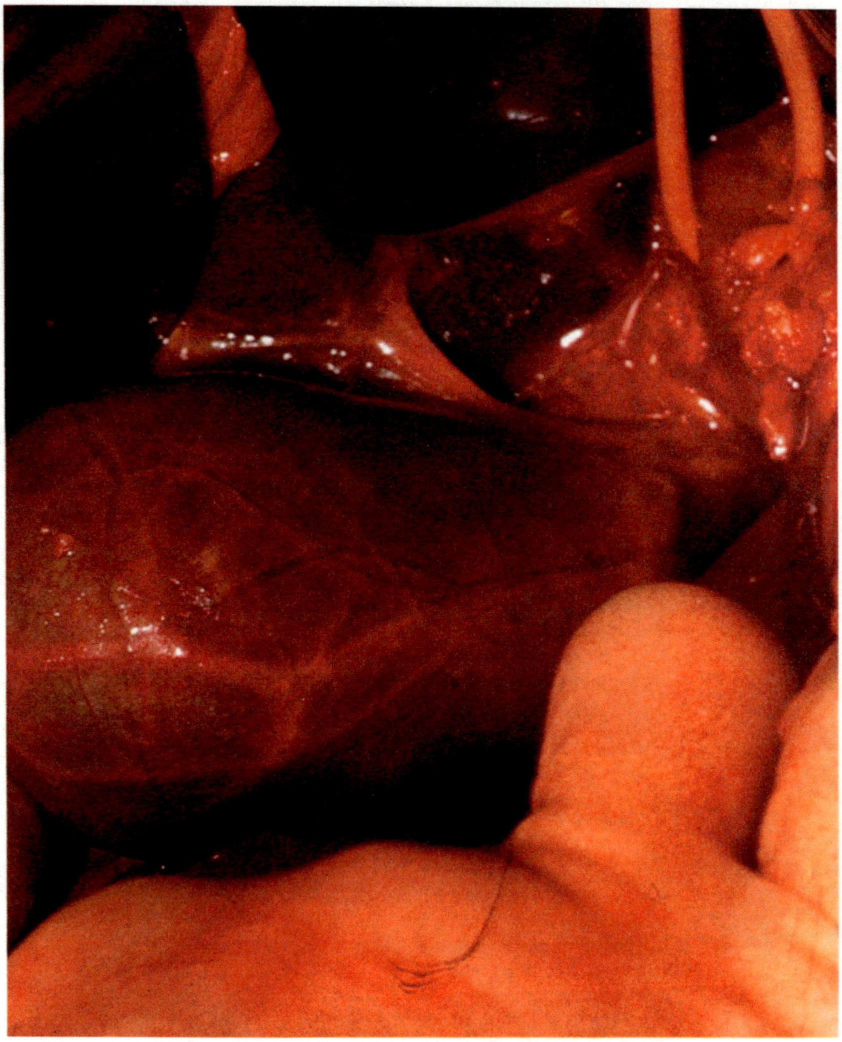

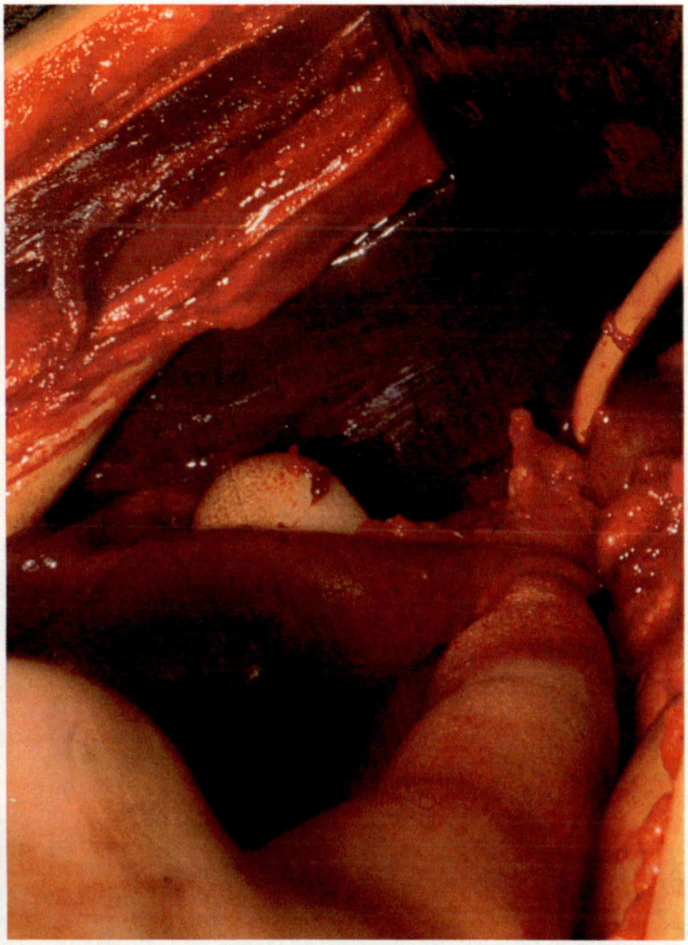

45

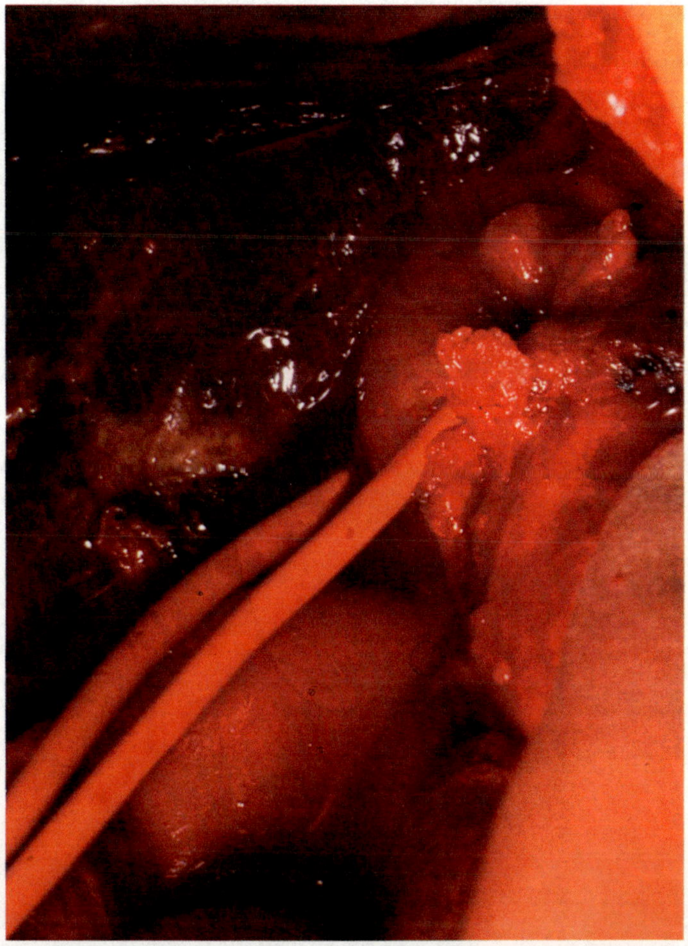

44 The cystic duct and artery are mobilised. The Hartmann's pouch area of the gallbladder is dissected free from the under surface of the liver.

45 The gallbladder is removed. Haemostasis is obtained along its bed; the common hepatic duct is exposed ready for division. It is only at this stage that the surgeon need feel committed to go on and perform a pancreatico-duodenectomy.

46 The common hepatic duct is divided close to the porta hepatis, so as to be well clear of malignant disease. In addition to the dilatation of the structure, the thick wall which develops after long-term obstruction facilitates suturing the biliary anastomosis. Bile is here being aspirated from the divided duct.

46

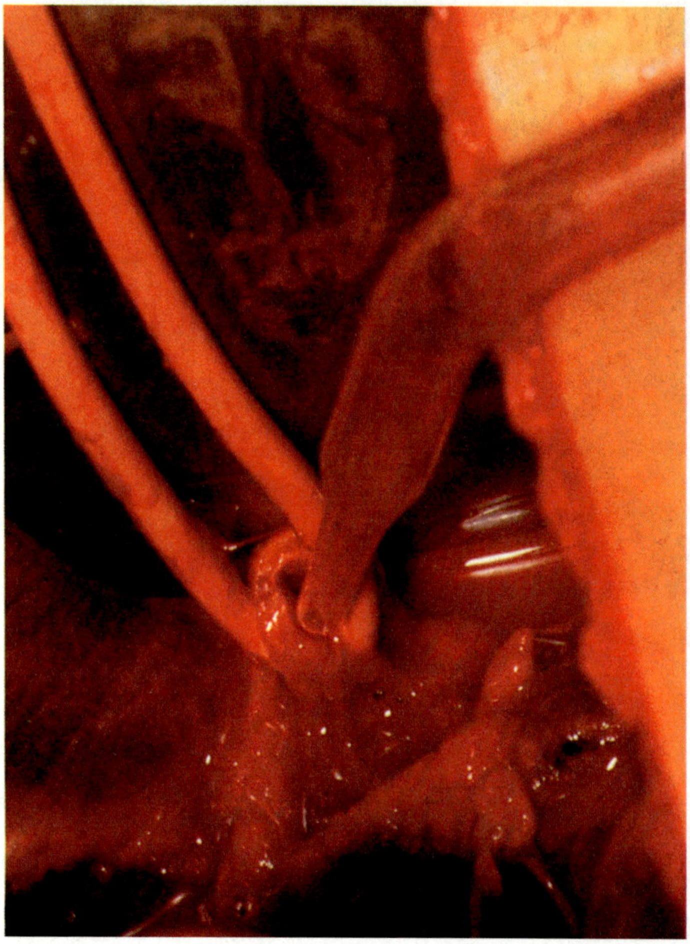

47

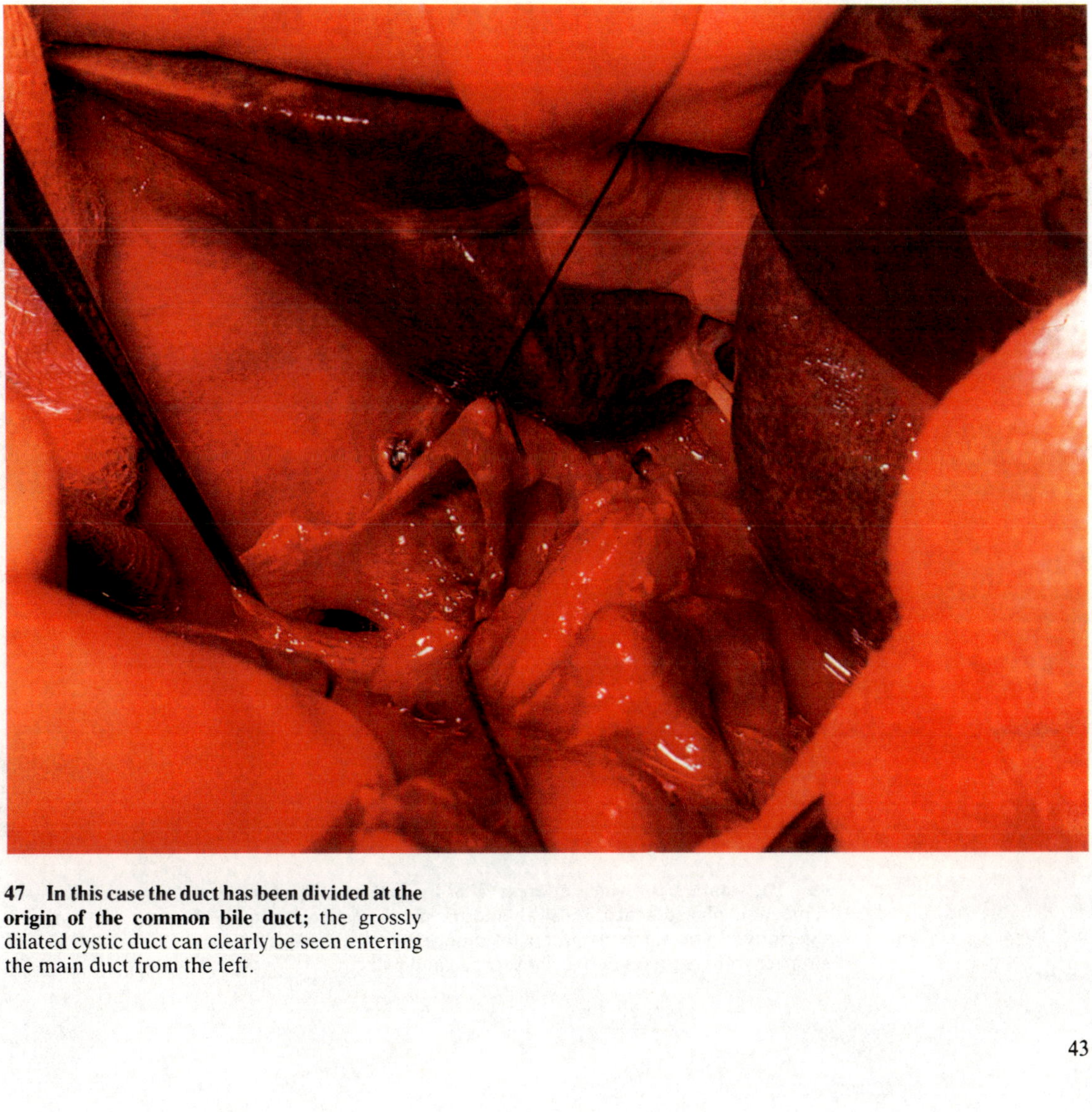

47 In this case the duct has been divided at the origin of the common bile duct; the grossly dilated cystic duct can clearly be seen entering the main duct from the left.

48

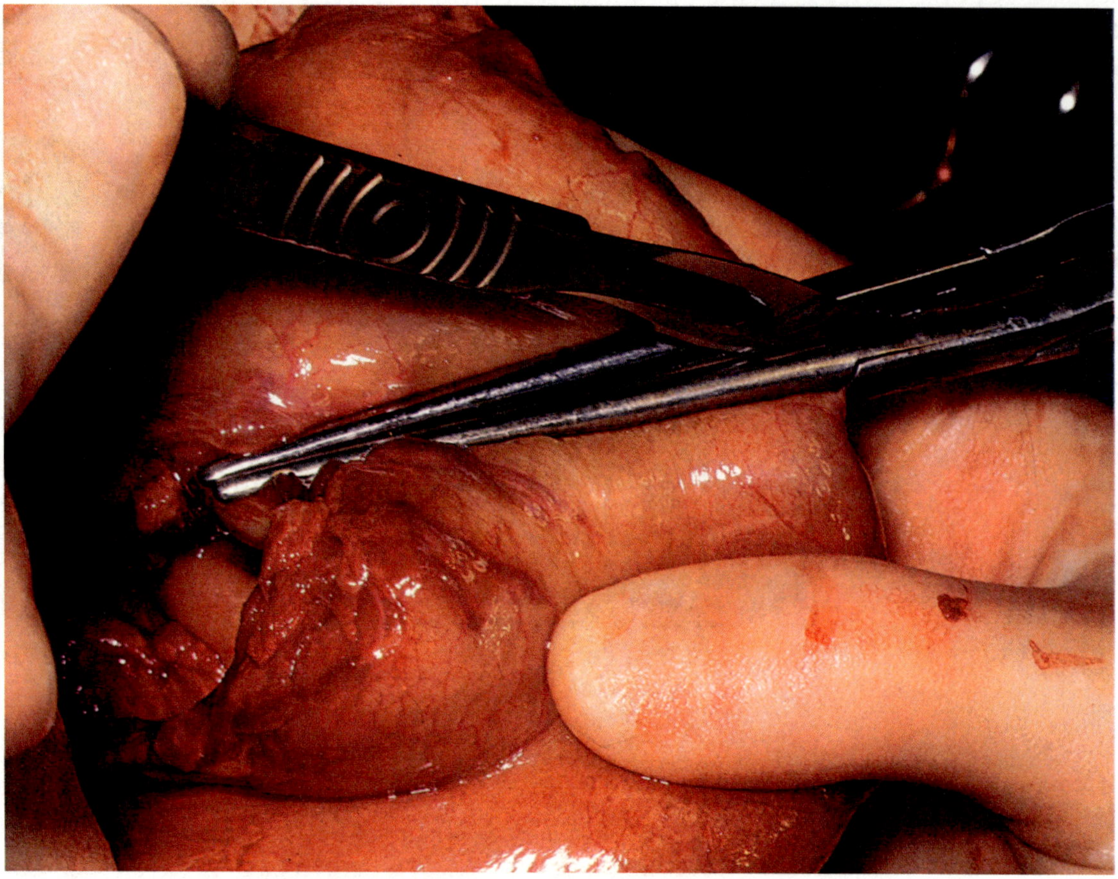

48 The stomach is divided at the level of the incisura. The proximal remnant is placed beneath a swab and the distal portion is retracted inferiorly. Some surgeons prefer to remove a greater portion of the stomach, others preserve the whole organ and pylorus.

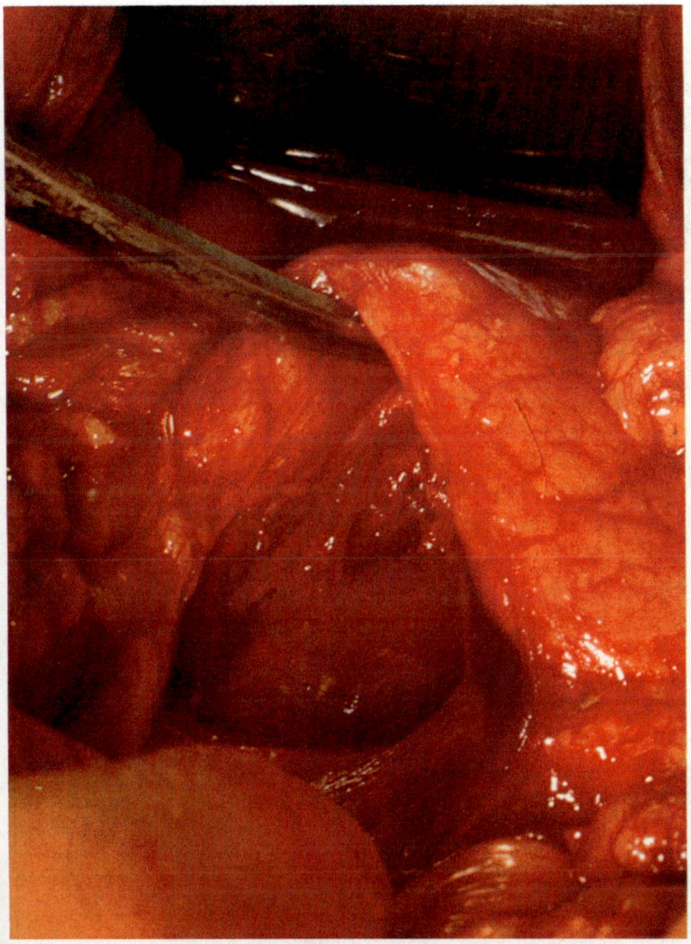

49 The pancreas is now ready for division and the main veins are well clear of the pancreas.

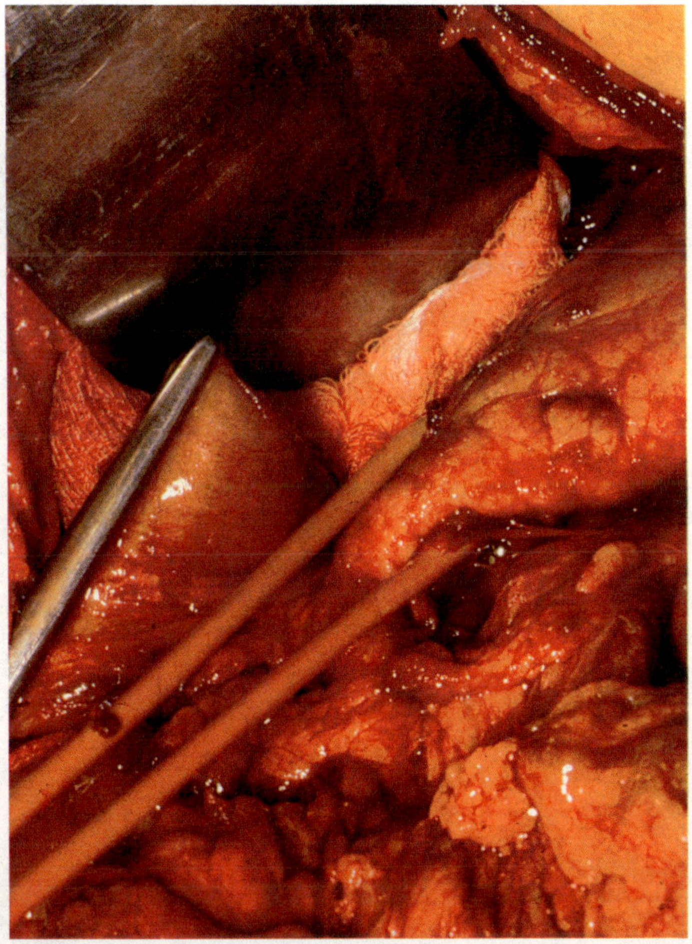

50

50 The gland is held firmly by a sling and the divided antrum is retracted clear of the field.

51 The neck of the pancreas can now be separated off the portal vein, and the pancreatic body is clear of the splenic vein for a distance of about 2 cm, to later facilitate performance of the pancreatic anastomosis.

51

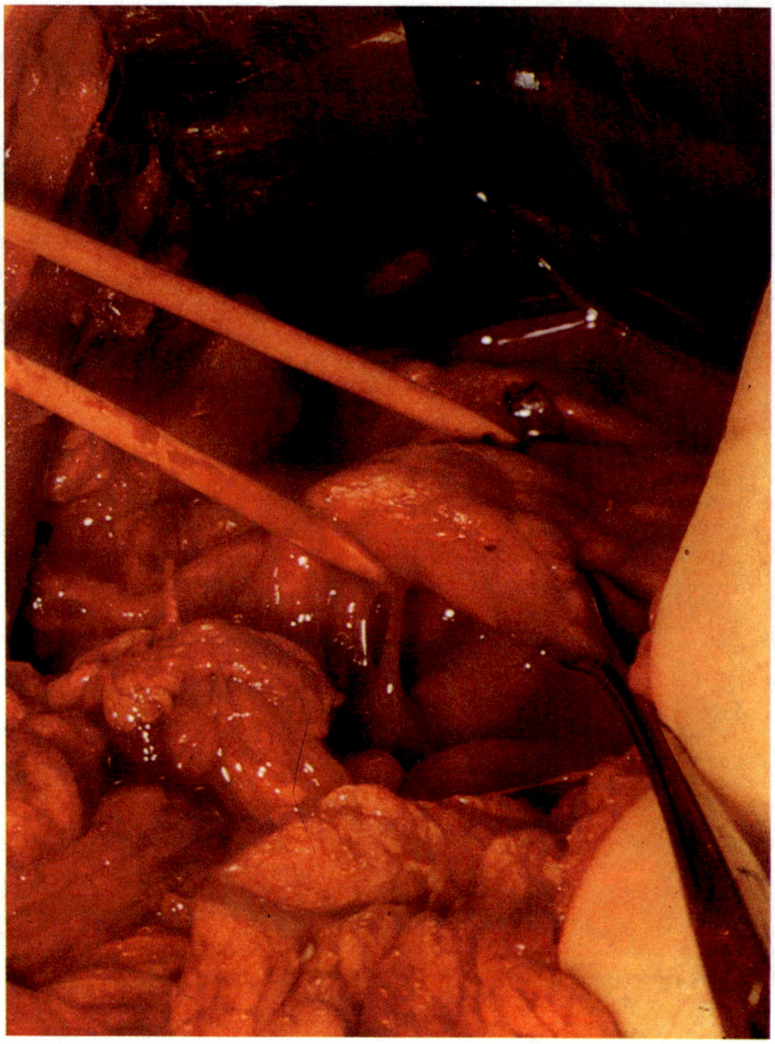

52

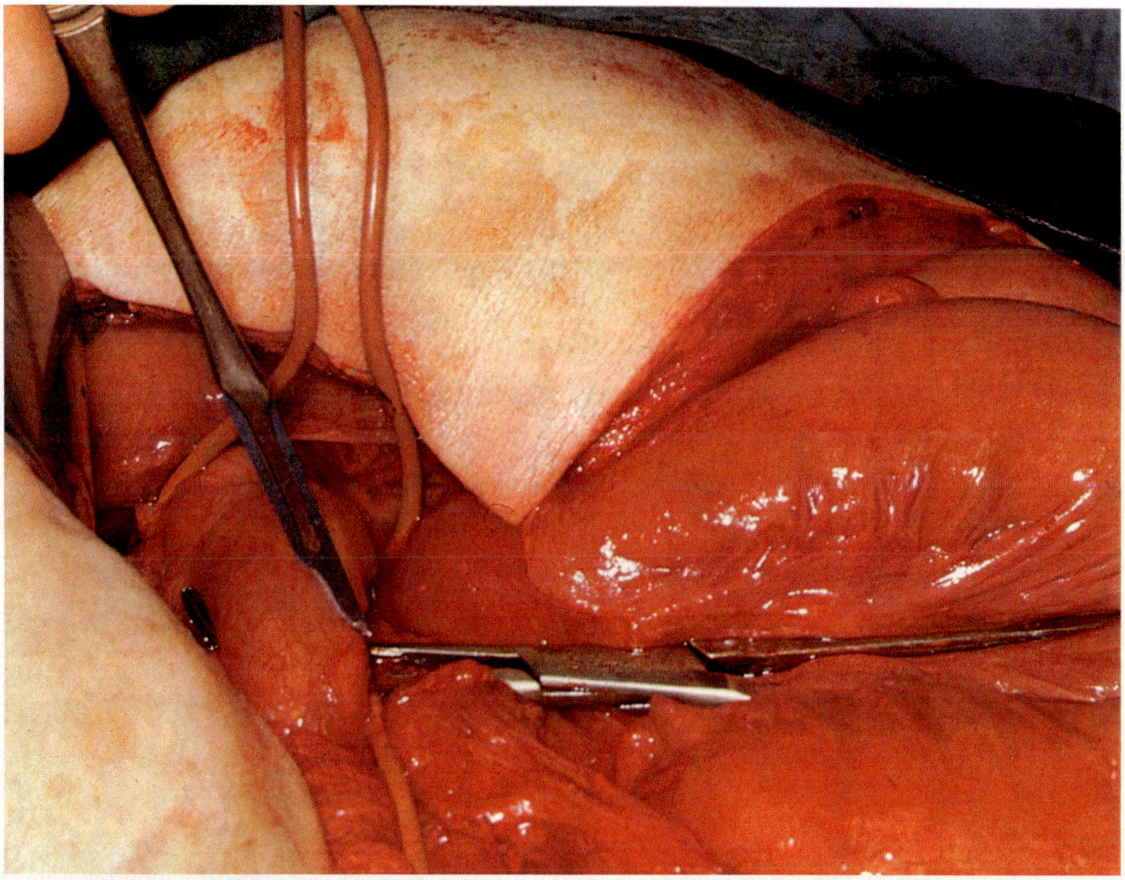

52 A pair of Lahey forceps is passed beneath the neck of the pancreas to protect the underlying vessels; the pancreas is divided using a fine scalpel.

53

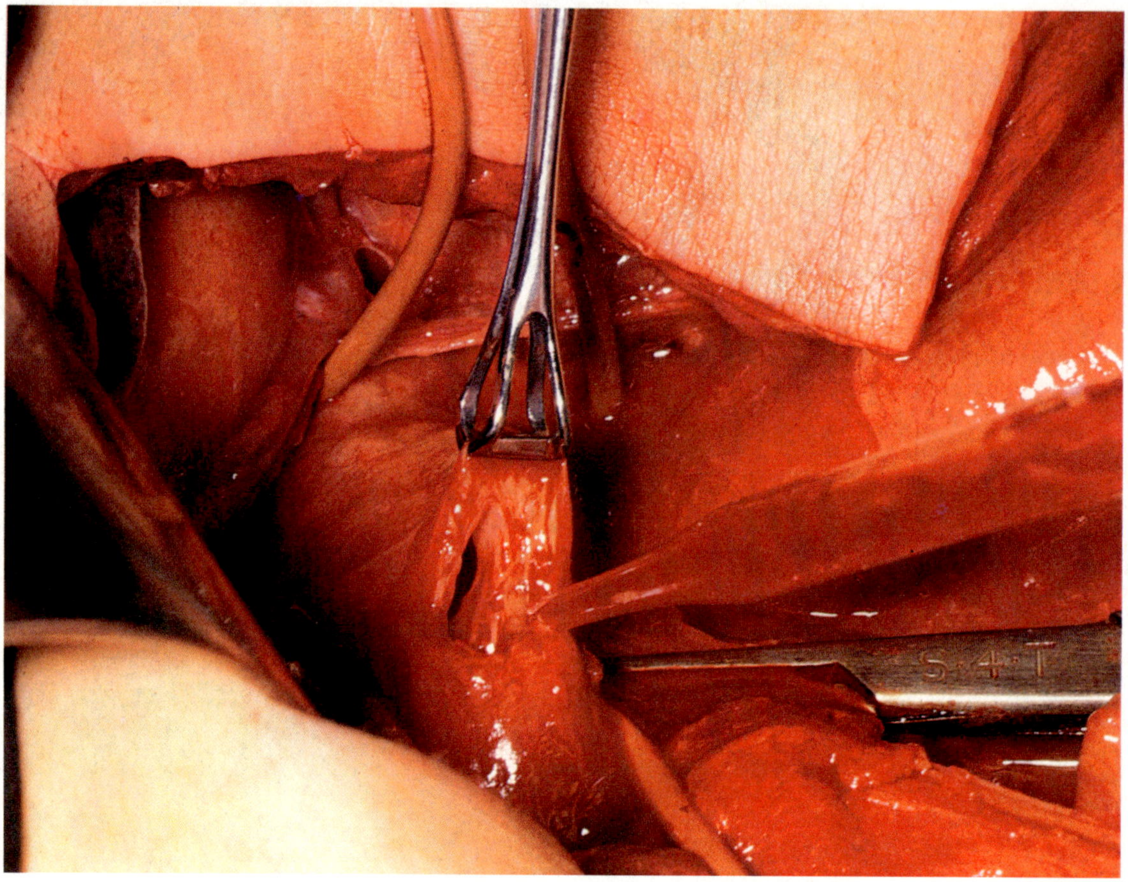

53 Partial division of the pancreas reveals a grossly dilated pancreatic duct, which is aspirated. A pair of Babcock's forceps is here gently applied to the outer edge of the pancreas.

54 **Division of the pancreas results in some bleeding from the divided surface;** a number of small vessels require ligation or diathermy. The divided bile duct can be seen above and in the left of the picture; the portal vein lies to the right.

54

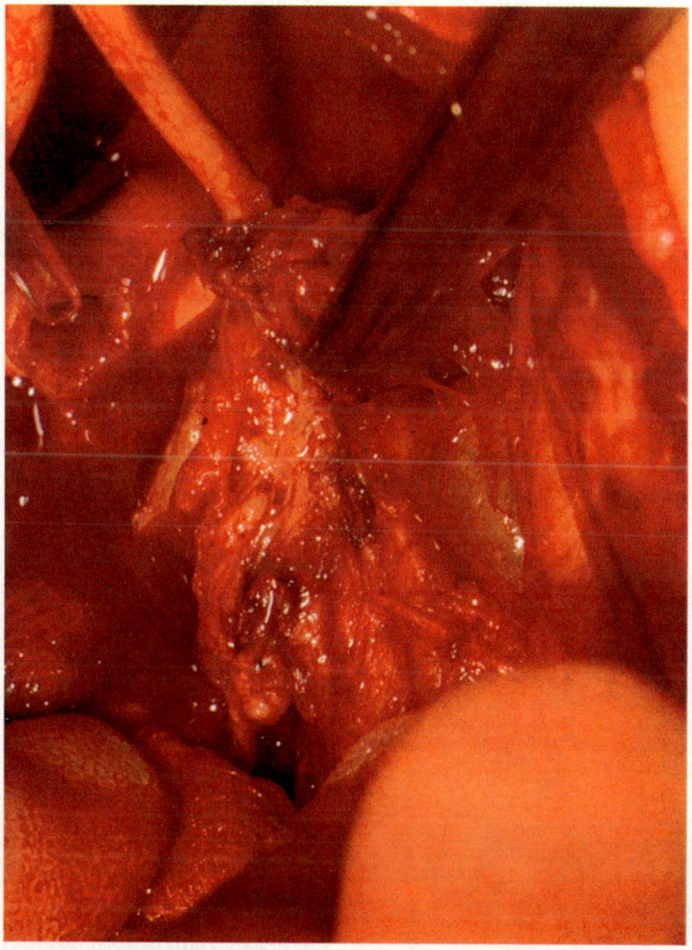

55

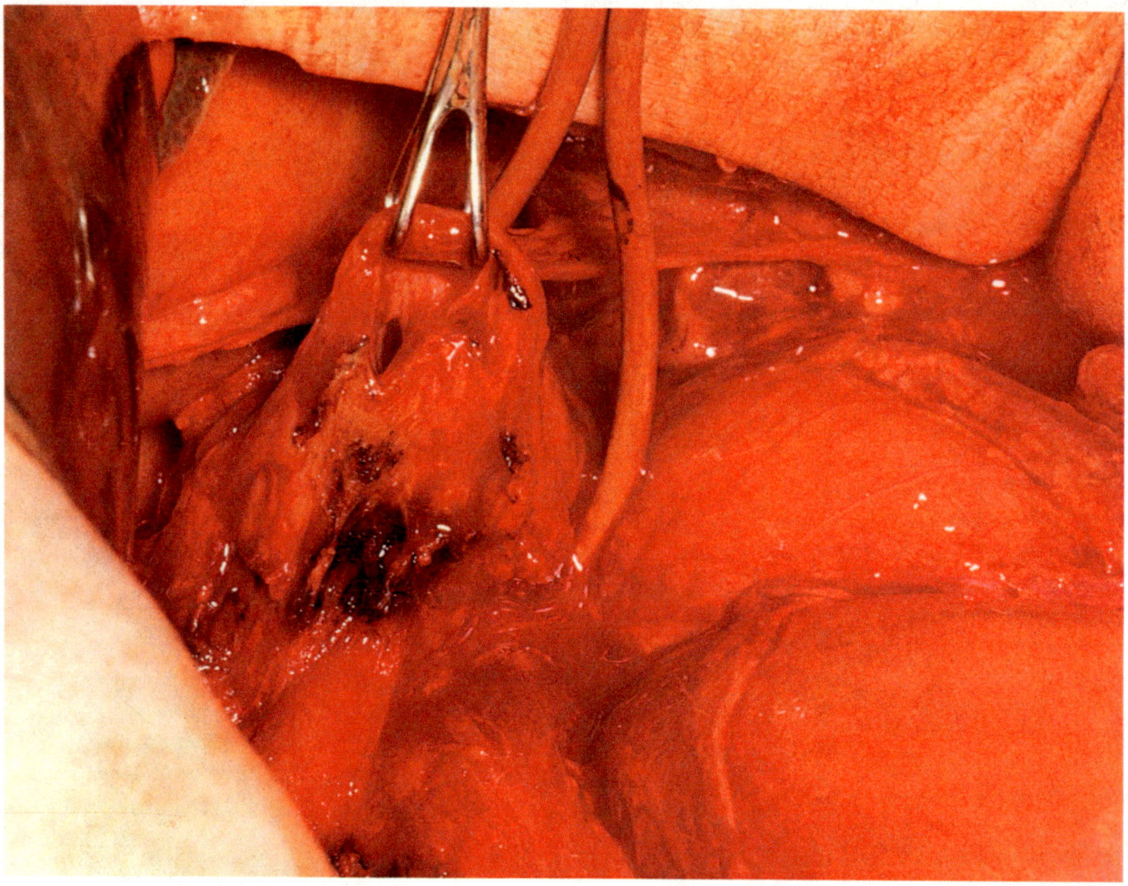

55 The duct of Wirsung is identified and dissected out, to project from the cut surface of the pancreatic body.

56 Division of the pancreas reveals the full length of the exposed superior mesenteric and portal veins. The splenic vein can here be seen coming across to enter the portal vein behind the stay suture.

56

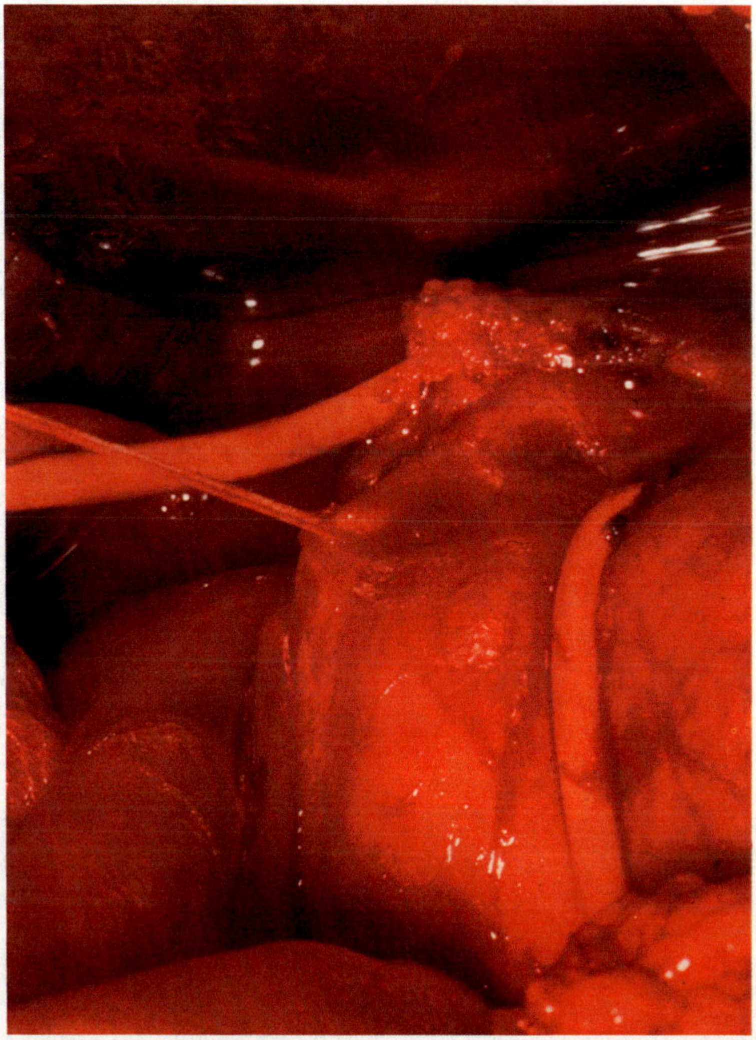

57

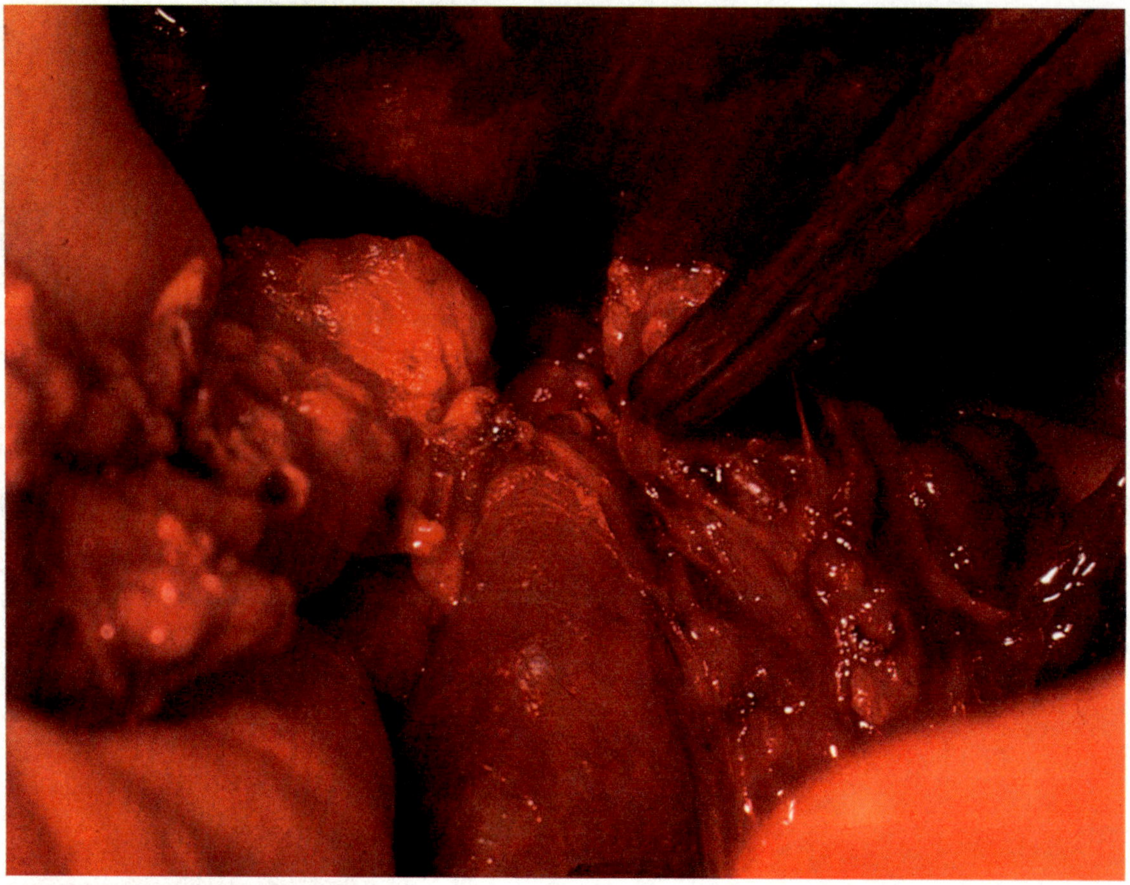

57 Those small veins running directly from the superior mesenteric vein into the head of the pancreas are next divided, and the head and uncinate process of the pancreas are separated from the portal vein.

58

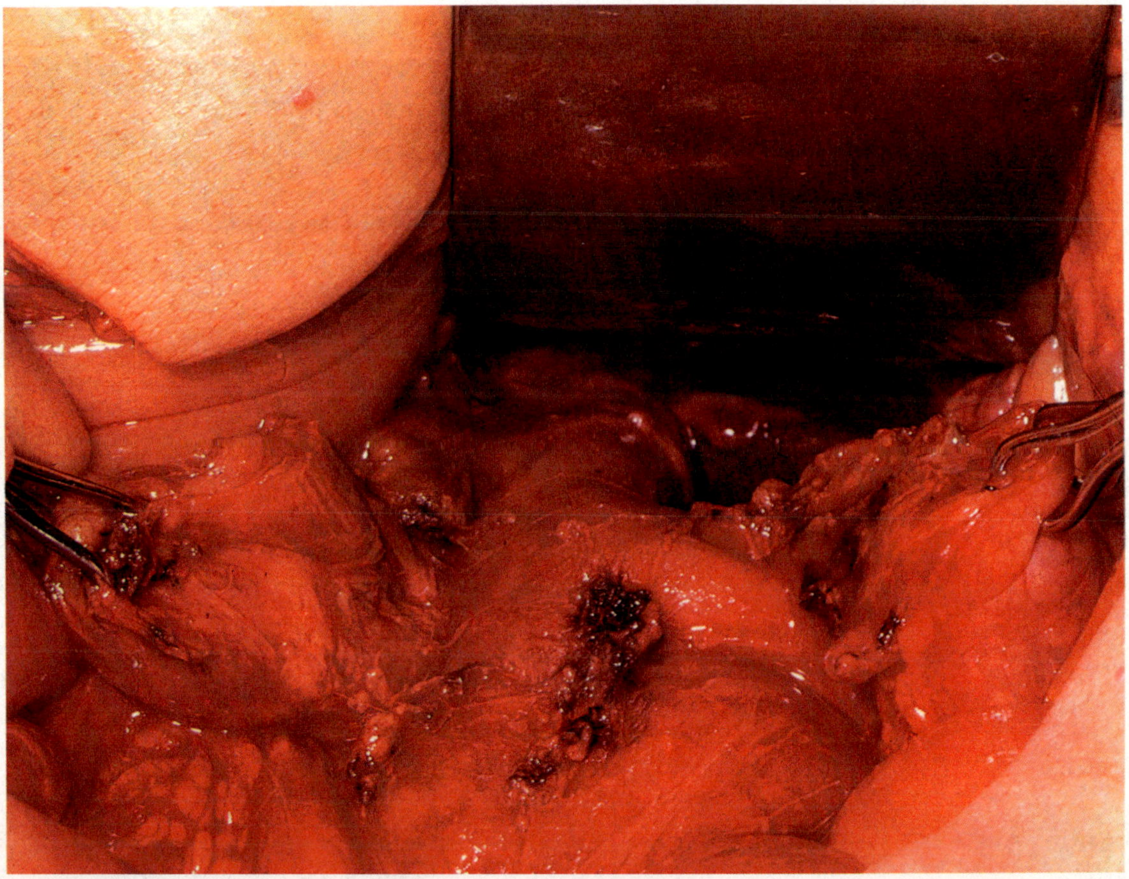

58 The divided edges of the pancreatic neck are here widely separated by traction on the two Babcock's forceps. The whole length of the superior mesenteric vein can be seen up to its junction with the splenic vein, beyond which the portal vein runs to the porta hepatis.

59 The jejunum is divided close to its origin, having mobilised the fourth part of the duodenum.

59

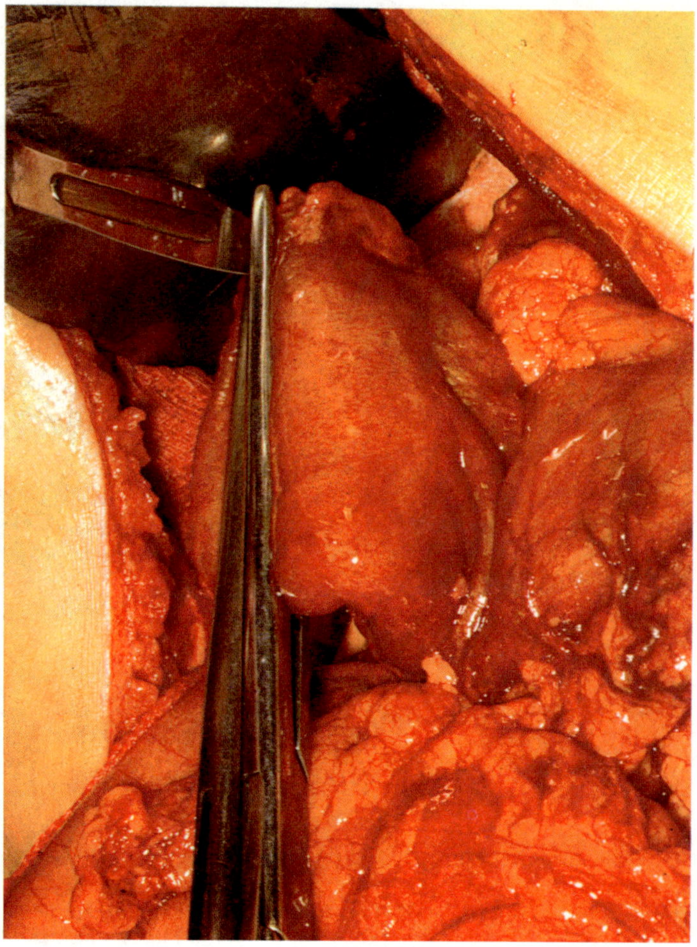

60

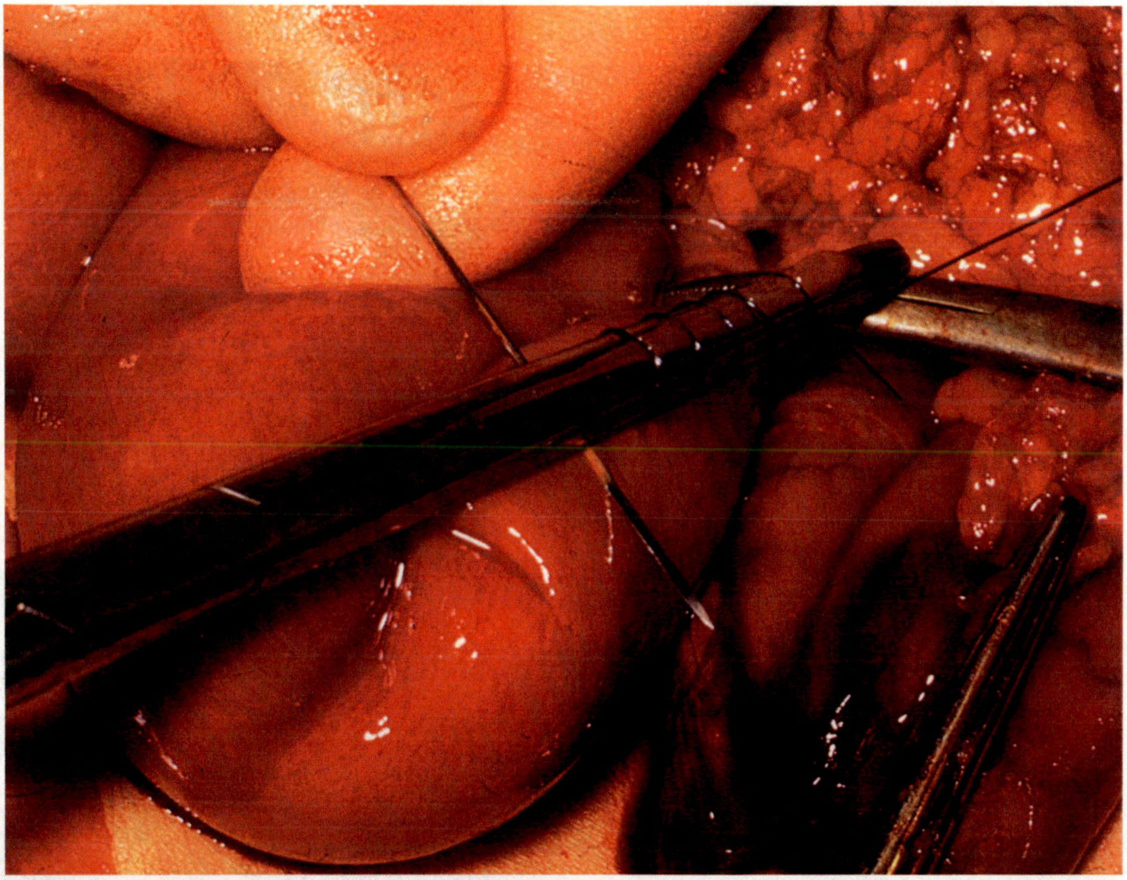

60 The distal end of the divided jejunum is then closed with two layers of suture material. It is convenient to oversew the stump with Prolene on a straight needle, to withdraw the clamp, and then perform the seromuscular closure.

61 **The completed two-layer jejunal closure** is shown here.

61

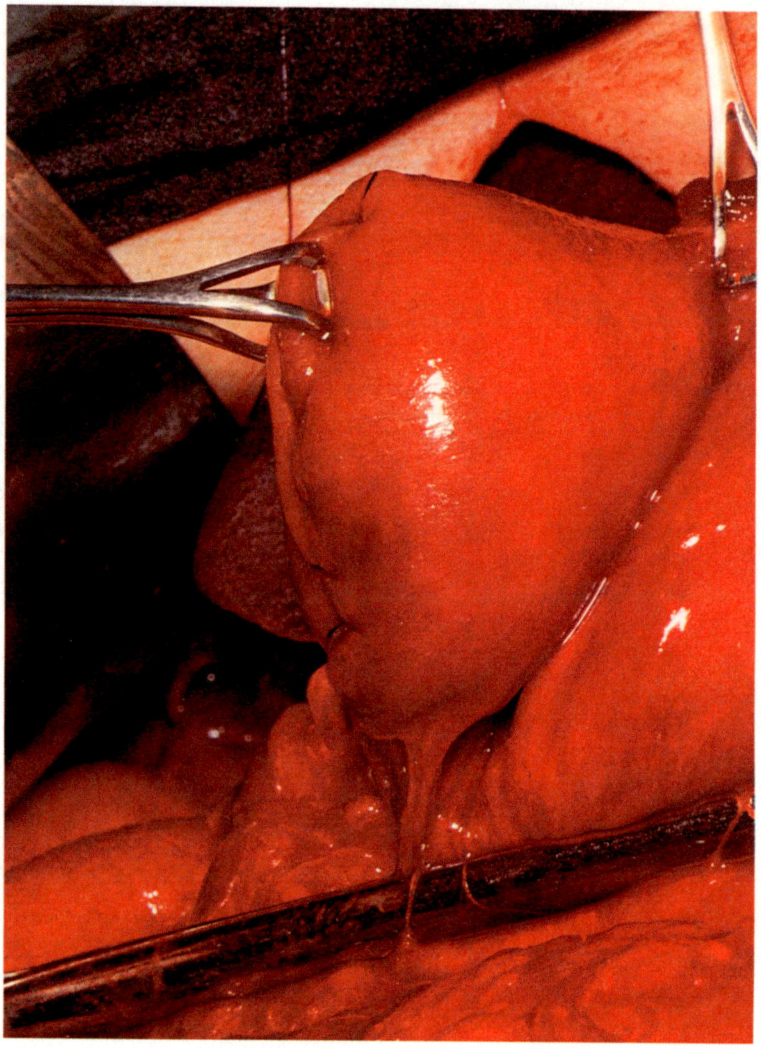

62 The uncinate process is the only remaining part of the specimen which remains fixed; this is now cleared from behind the main blood vessels, chiefly by blunt dissection. The specimen which consists of the distal stomach, the whole duodenum, the first few centimetres of jejunum, the gallbladder, the whole common bile duct, and the head and neck portion of the pancreas are now removed.

62

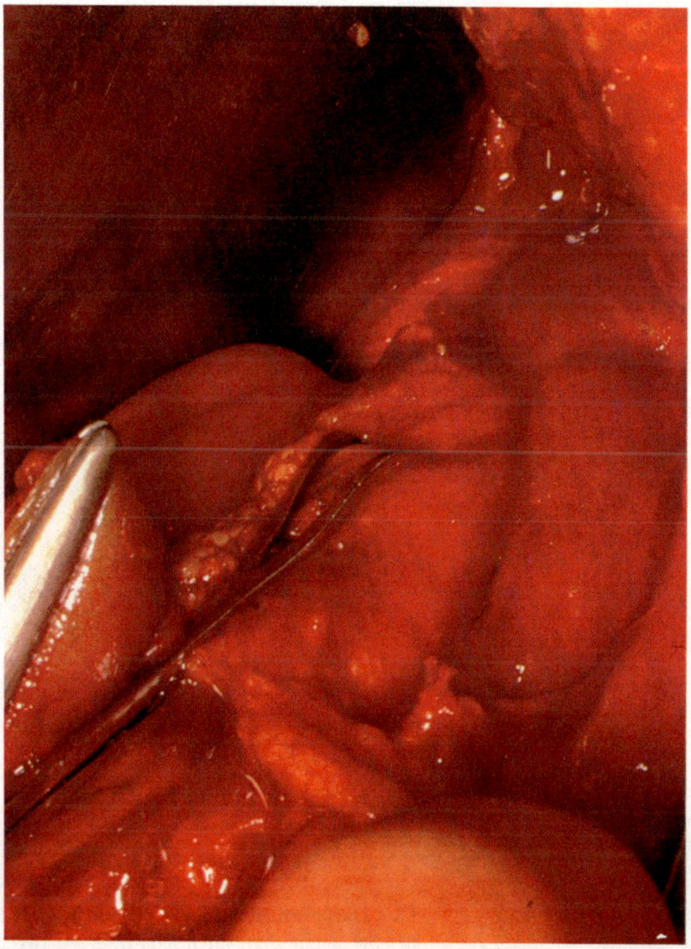

63

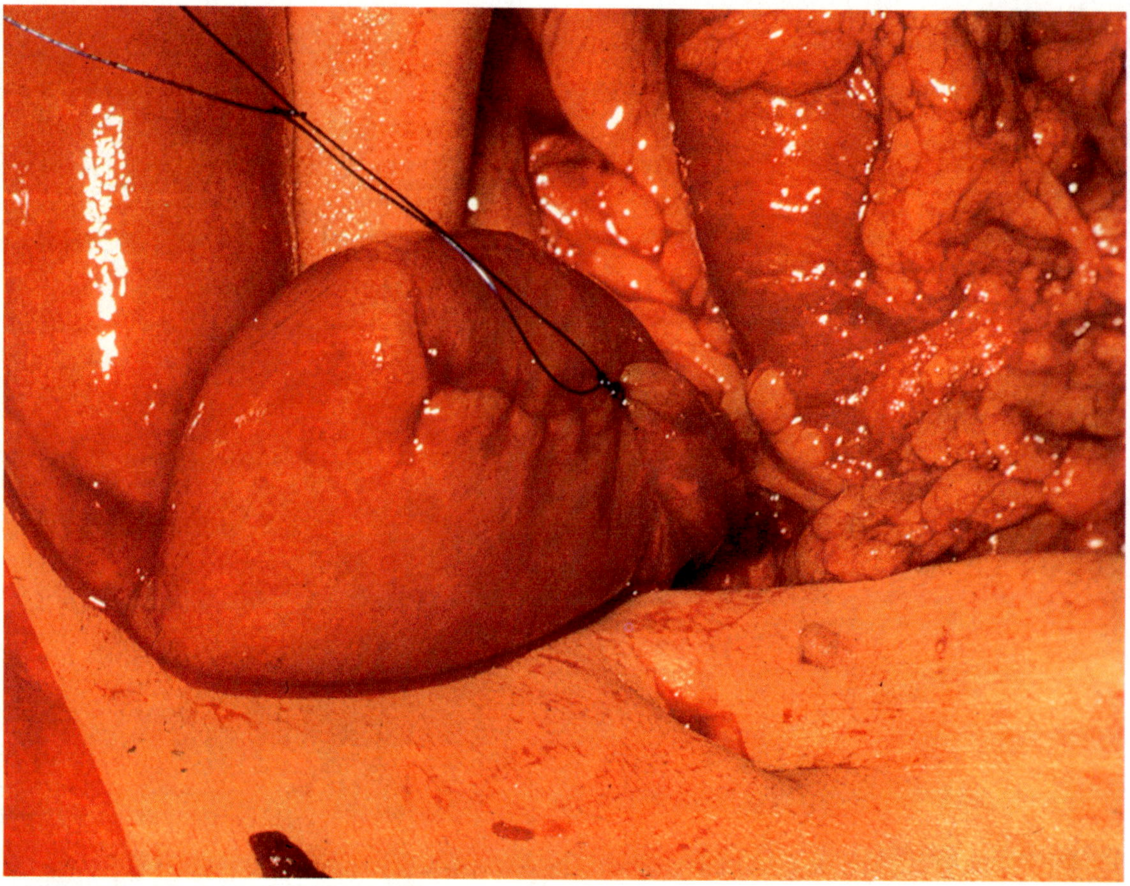

63 The proximal jejunum is lifted in front of the transverse colon to lie in the right hypochondrium, close to the liver. An antecolic anastomosis is preferred, because recurrence rates are high; local invasion may be less likely to produce obstruction of either the jejunum or the stomata, if an antecolic anastomosis is performed.

64

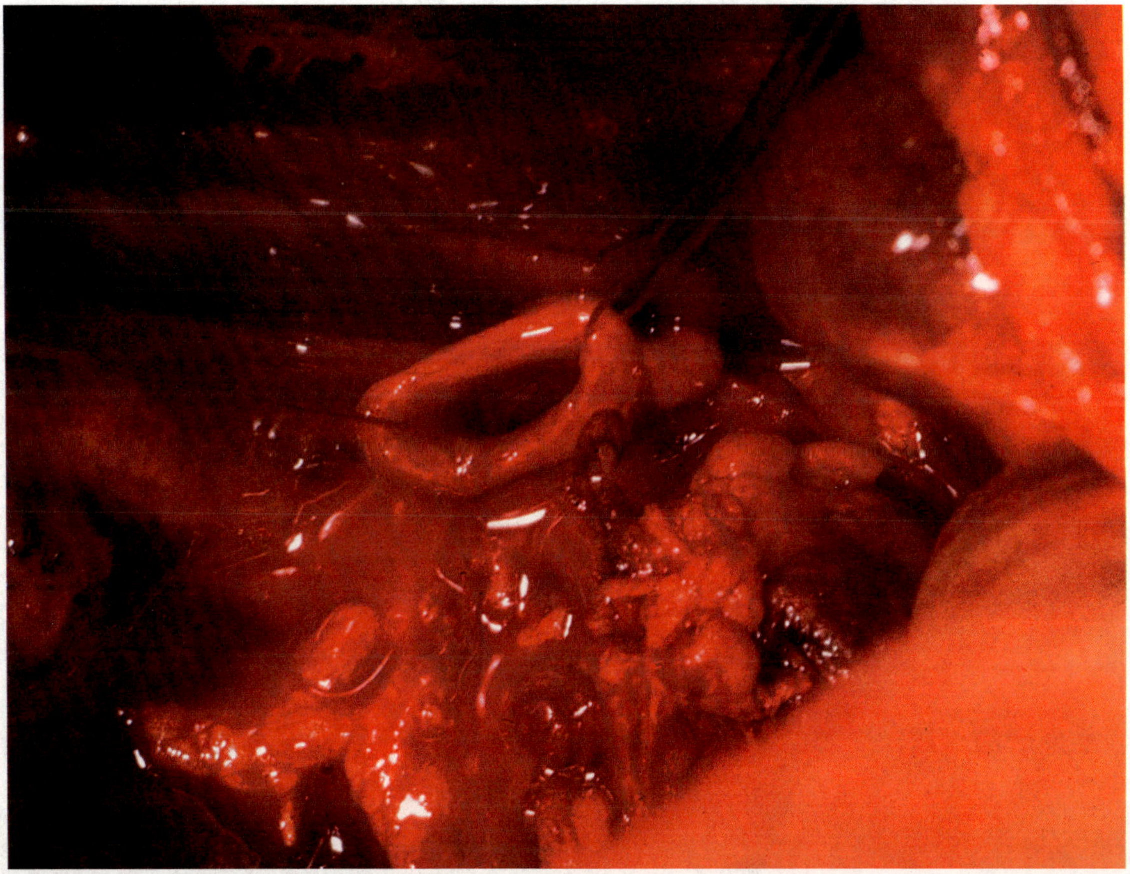

64 Two-stay sutures are next placed through the lateral edges of the divided common hepatic duct, before performing the first anastomosis between this duct and the jejunum.

65

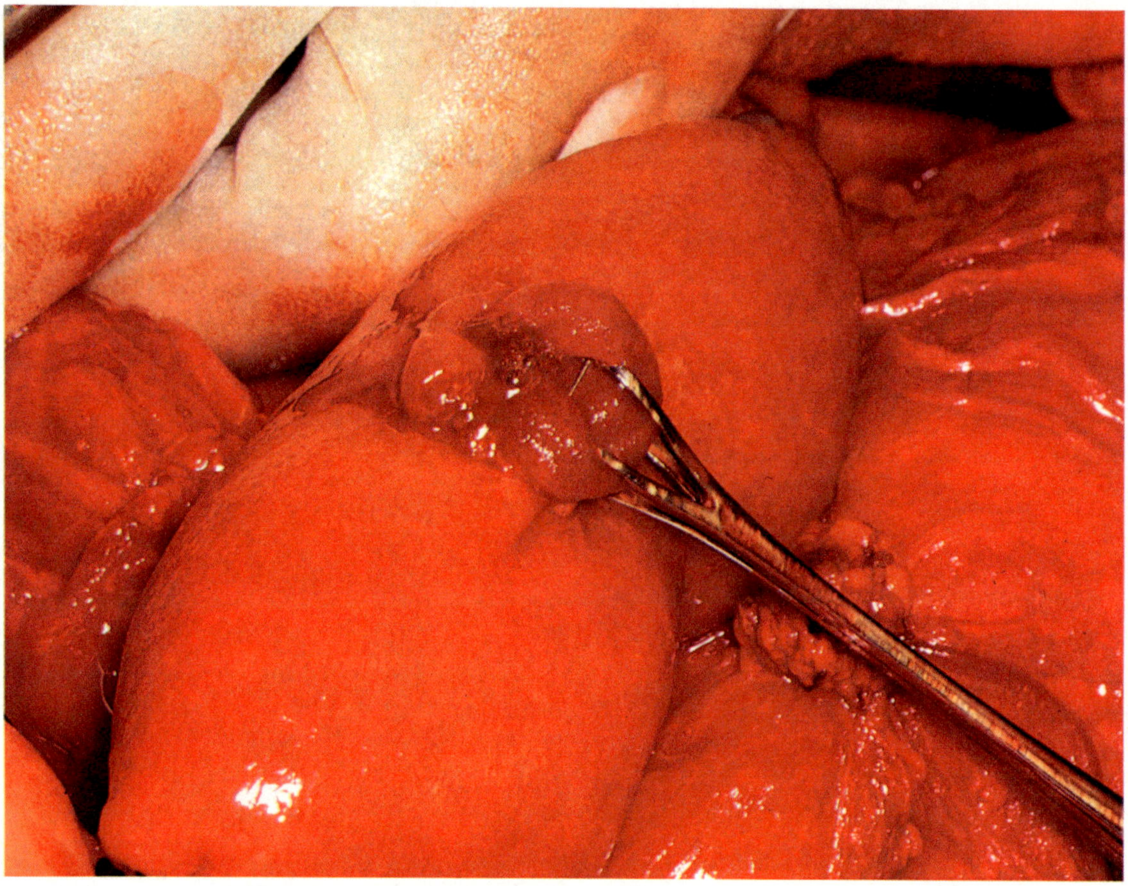

65 About 4 cm from the closed end of the jejunum an incision is made in its antimesenteric border and the mucosa is everted. This incision need only be a few millimetres long, because it dilates very easily. It is a mistake to make too large a stoma.

66
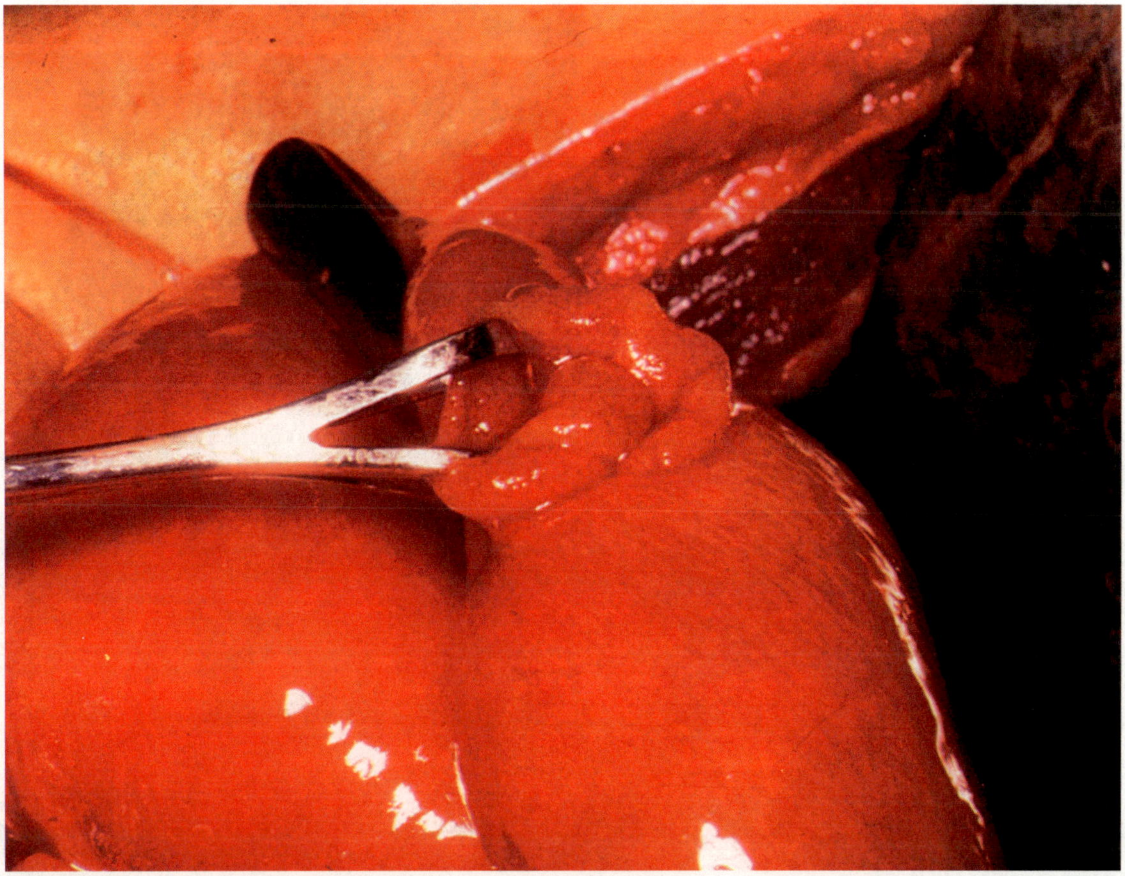

66 A pair of Babcock's forceps is placed along the anterior wall of the anastomosis; a light occlusion clamp is placed across the jejunal loop to prevent spillage of intestinal contents, and to reduce bleeding.

67

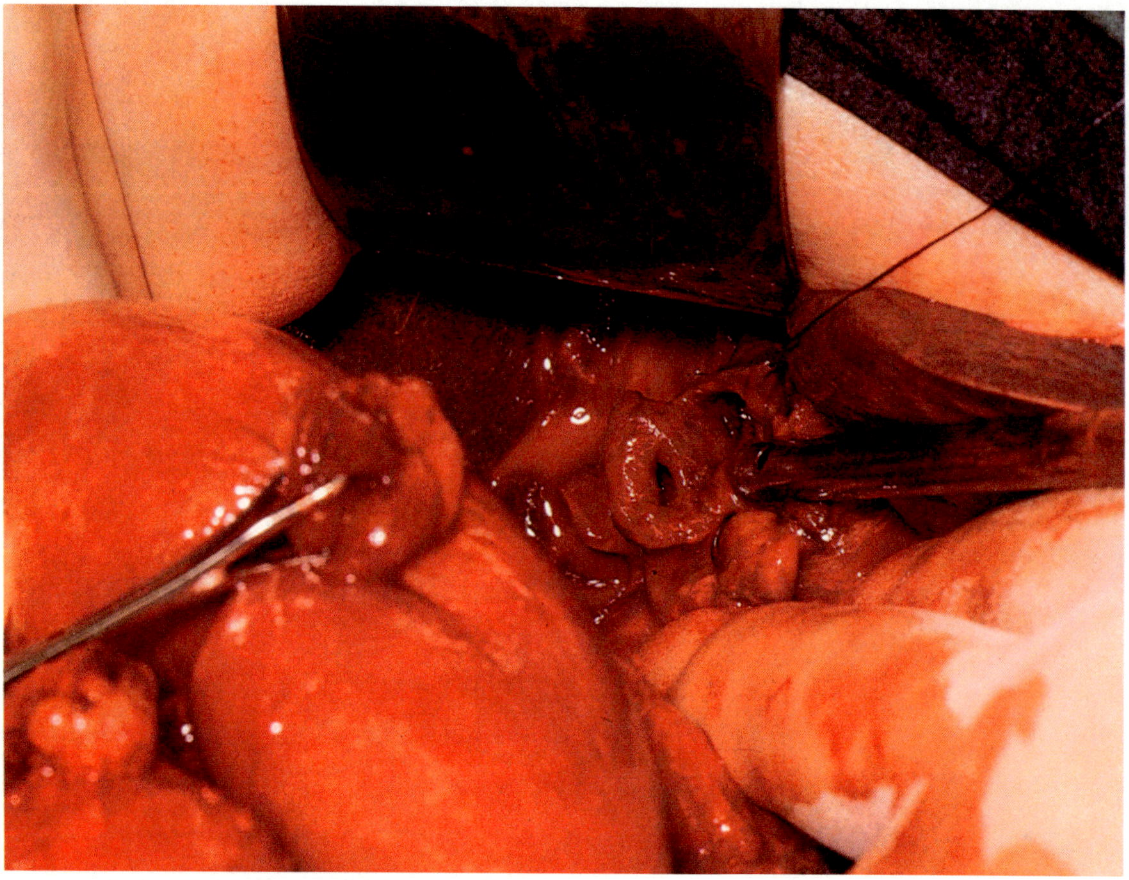

67 The jejunal opening is next placed about 3 cm or 4 cm from the divided common bile duct, so that the anastomosis can be performed. It is of utmost importance to check that the jejunal loop reaches the porta hepatis easily, and will lie there without tension.

68

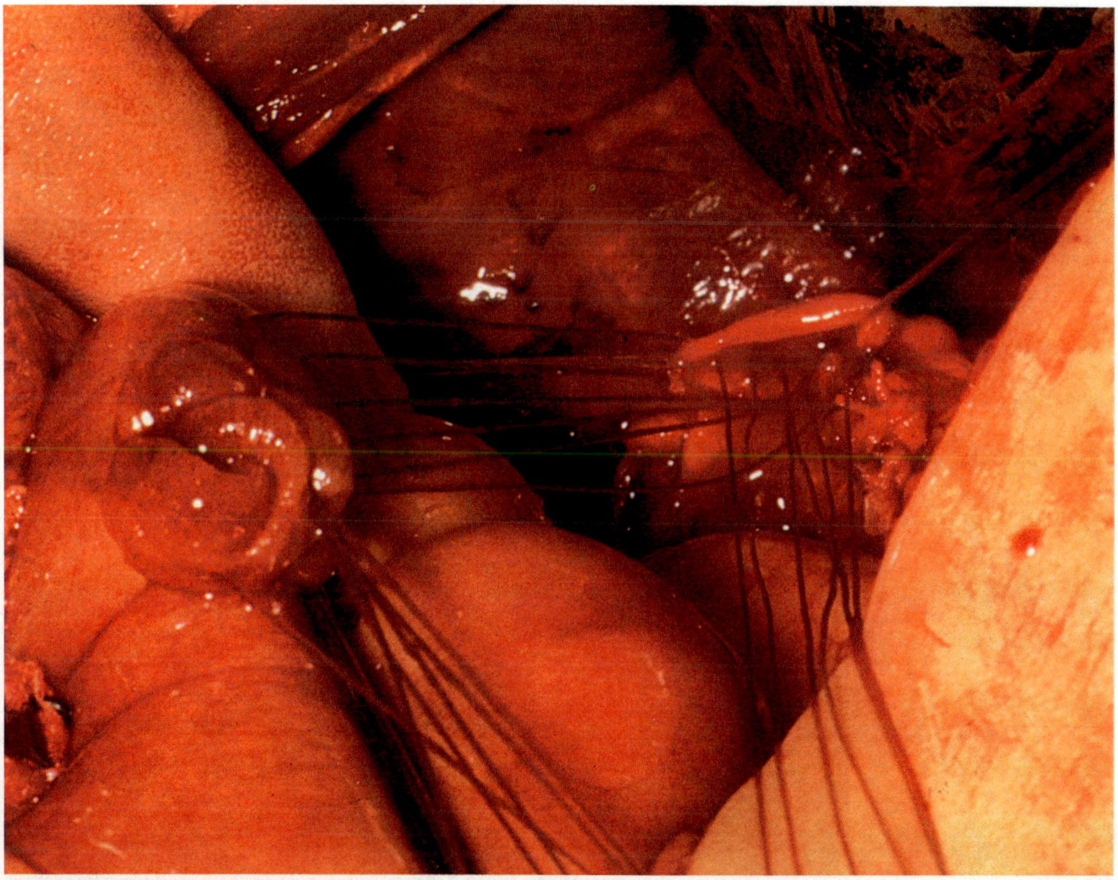

68 The posterior layer of the anastomosis is performed by placing individual catgut sutures through the full thickness of the jejunum and the common hepatic duct in turn. Numbered artery forceps are useful in preventing twisting or the overlapping of sutures. Approximately six sutures are used for the posterior layer, though this does vary according to the diameter of the hepatic duct.

69

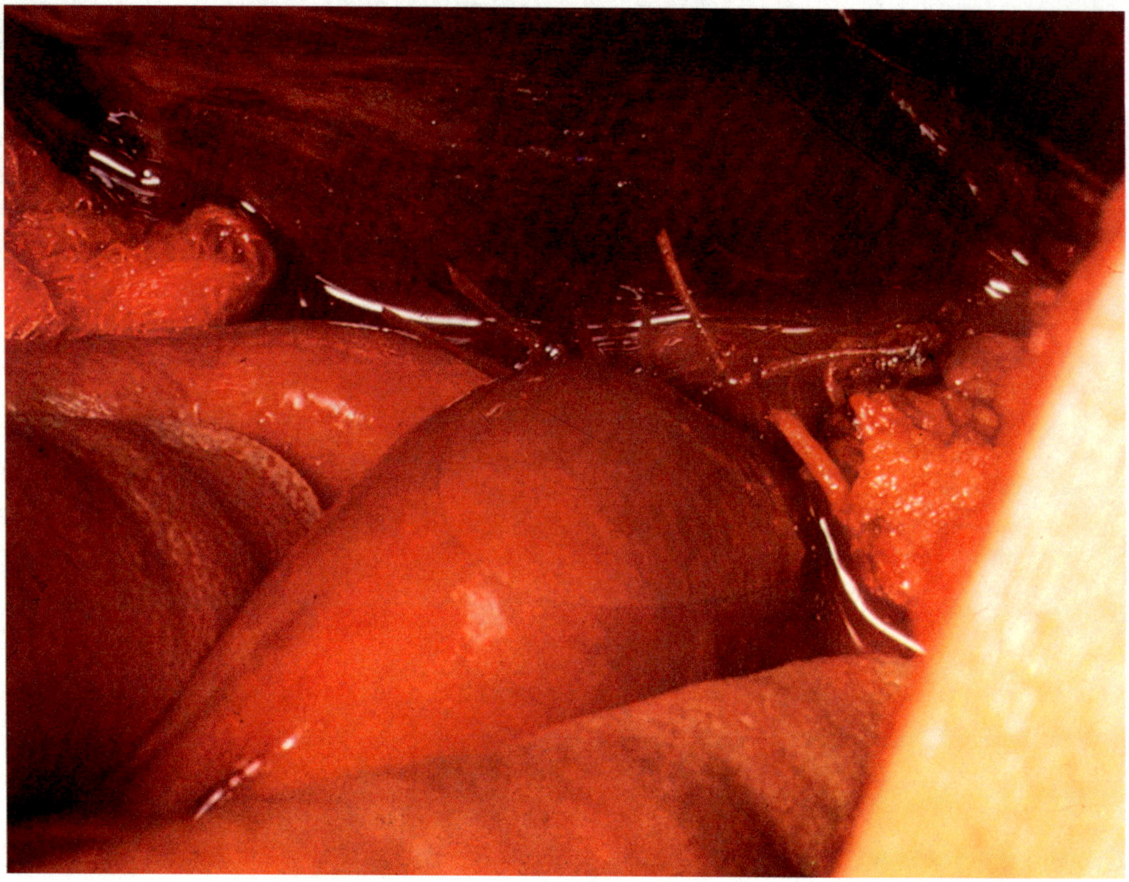

69 The jejunum is slid along these sutures and the posterior layer of the anastomosis is tied. The anterior layer of full thickness sutures is next inserted in similar manner; these are ligated and finally cut.

70

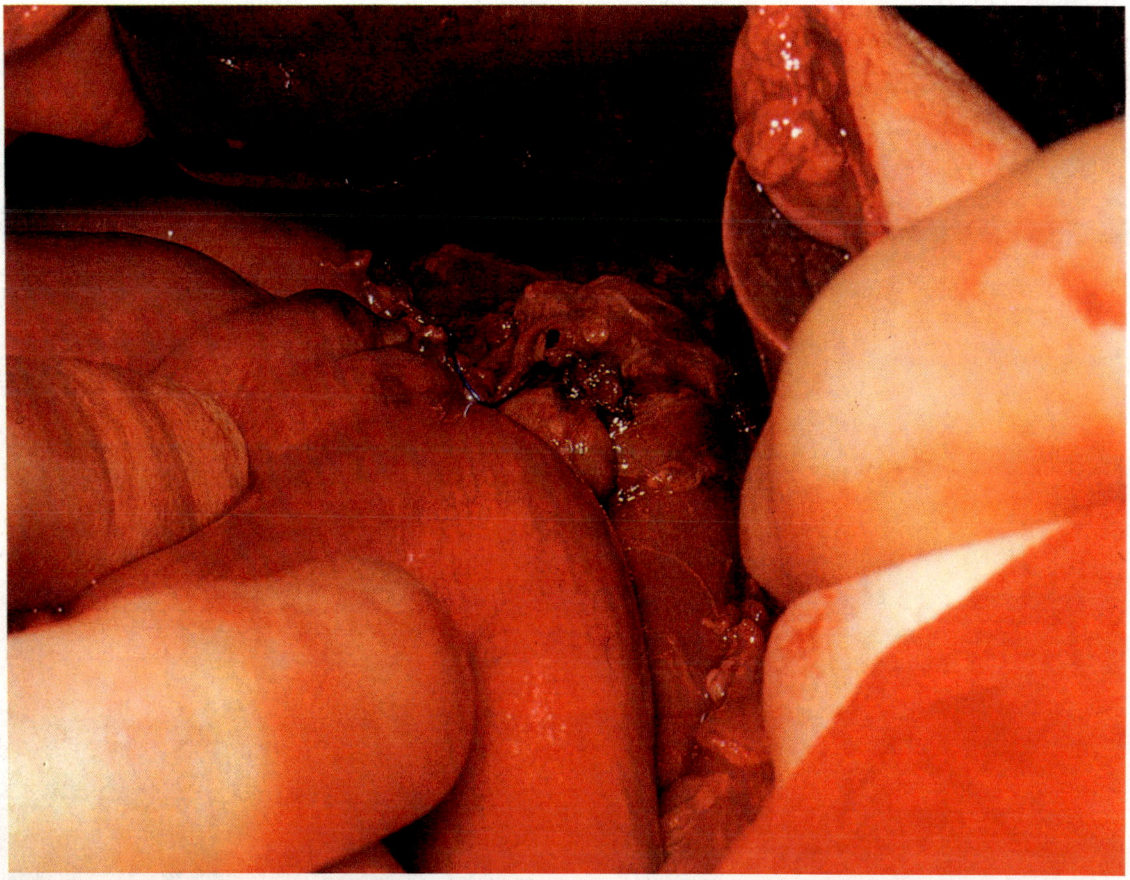

70 One layer of sutures inserted in this way, without tension, is probably adequate for this anastomosis, but a second layer may be used to reinforce the seromuscular layer, as shown here.

71 Light occlusion clamps are placed on a loop of jejunum and across the body of the pancreas, close to the resection line. The posterior layer of the pancreatic anastomosis is performed suturing the seromuscular layers of the jejunum to the outer space of the body of the pancreas with a continuous suture.

71

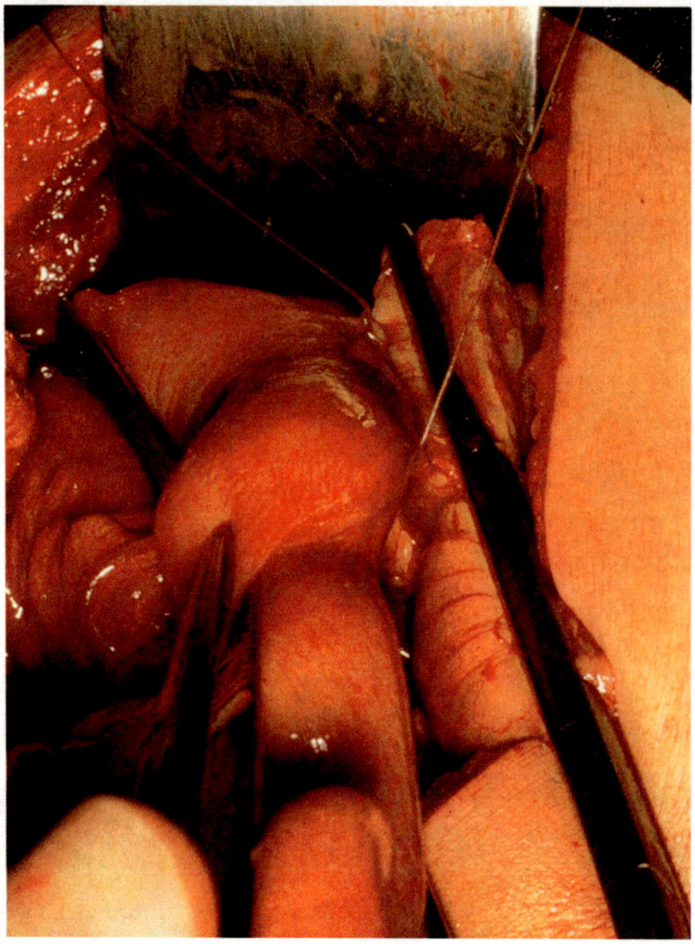

72

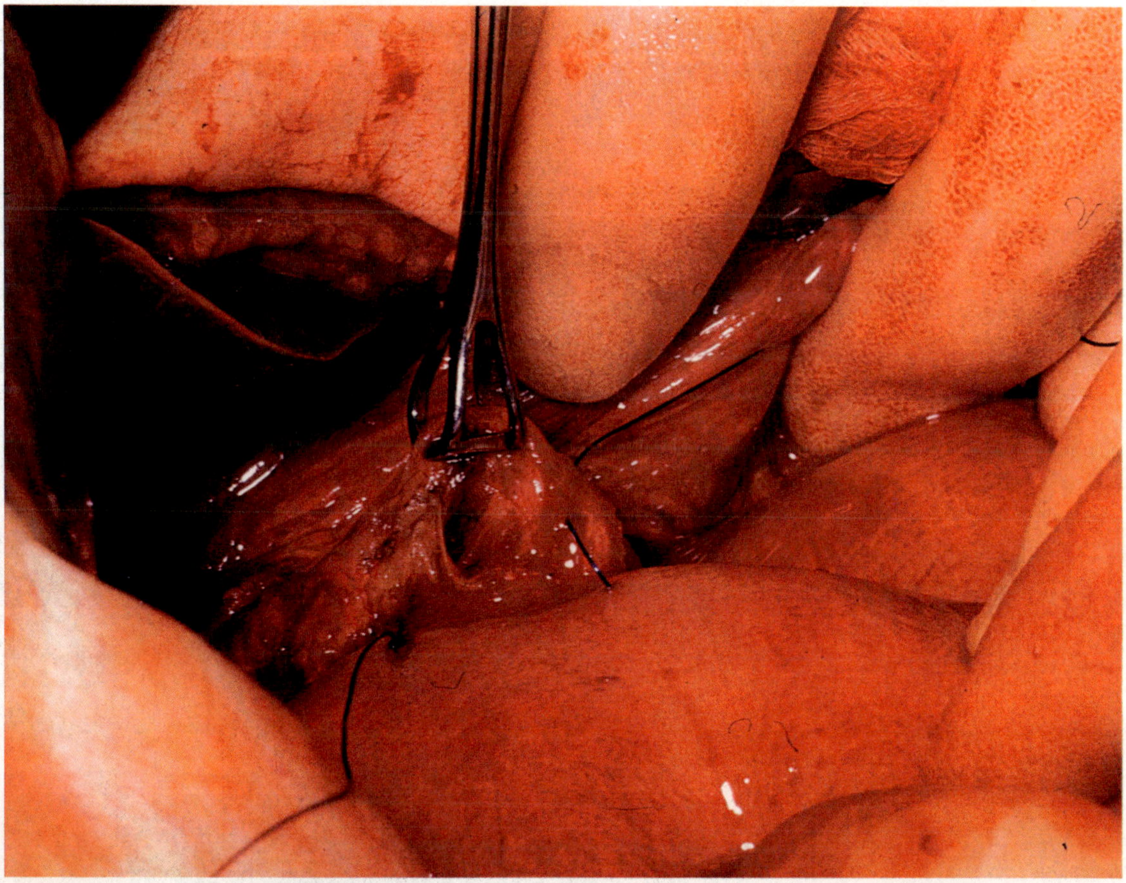

72 The posterior layer of the pancreatico-jejunal anastomosis is shown here. This patient suffers from marked dilatation of the pancreatic duct.

73

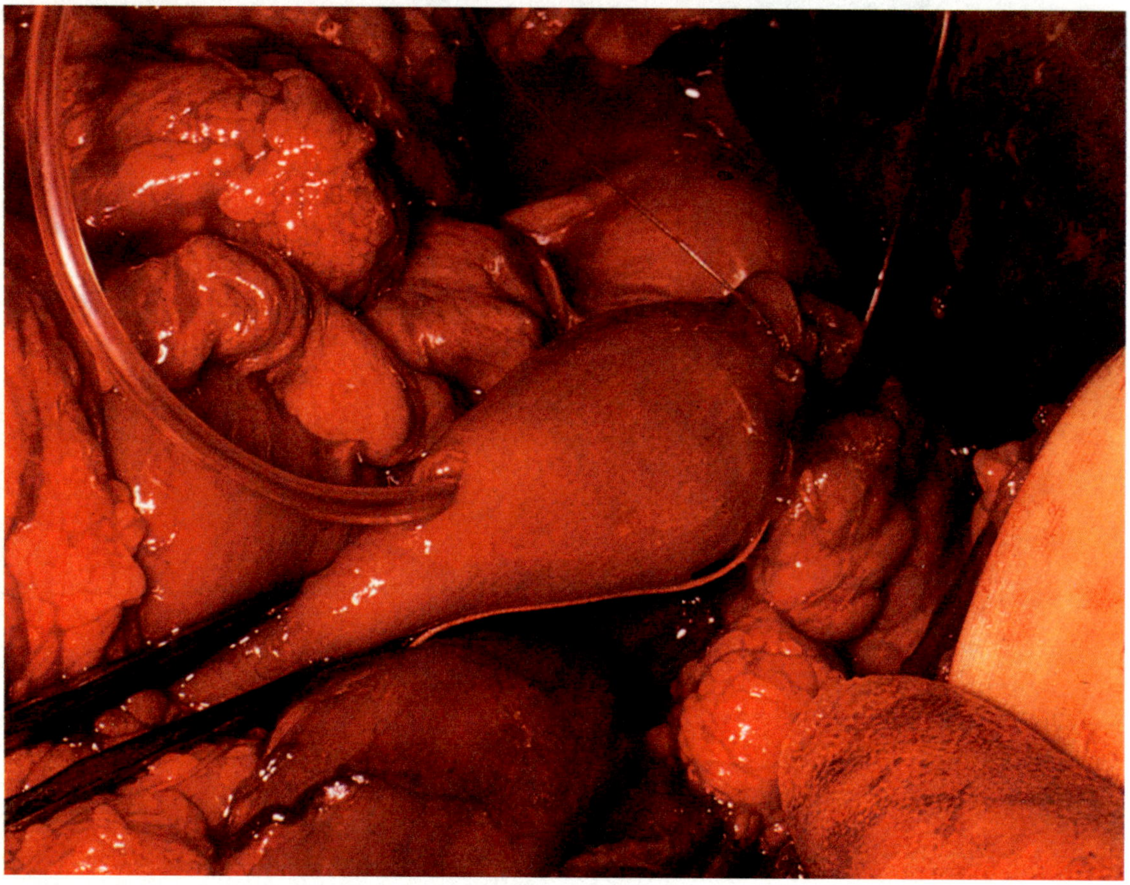

73 A fine Portex cannula is inserted through the jejunum, approximately 5 cm distal to the anastomosis and through a small hole in the jejunal mucosa across the anastomosis. Its tip lies about halfway along the pancreatic duct. The duct mucosa and pancreatic mucosa are anastomosed using catgut.

74

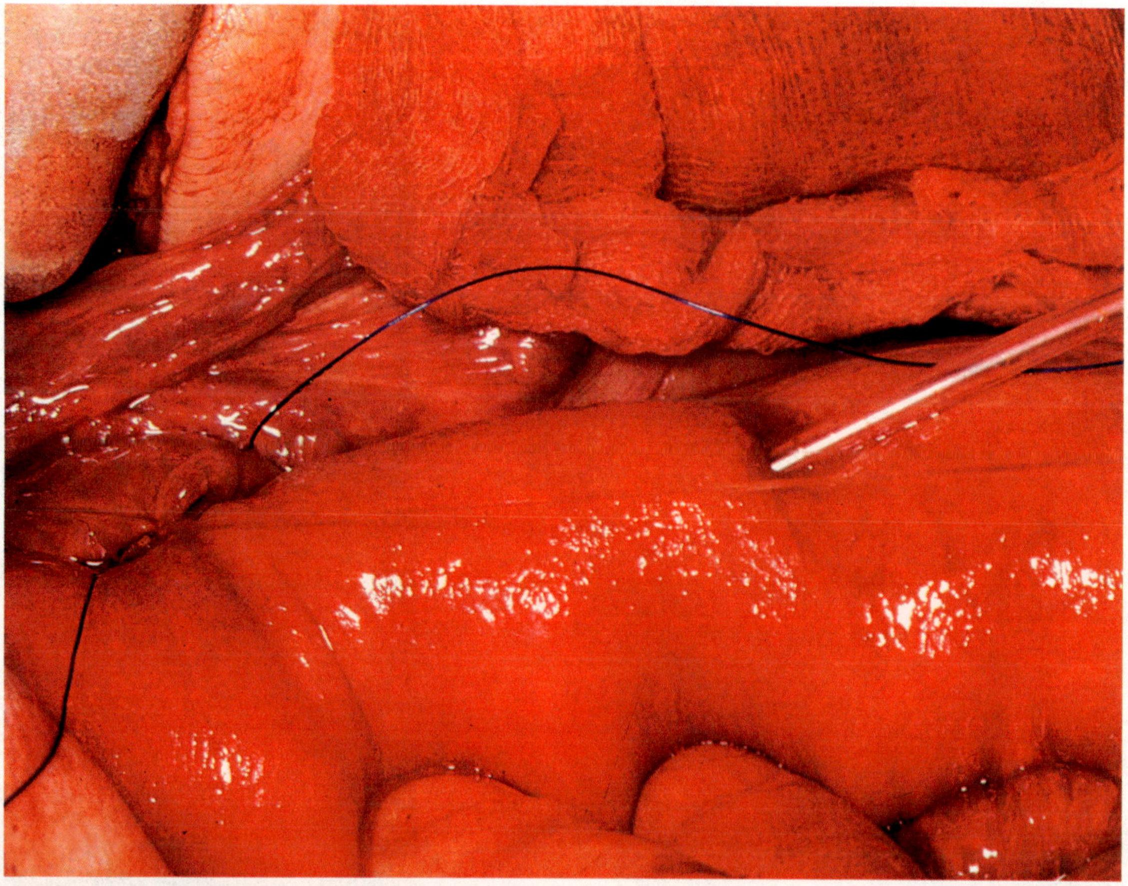

74 The anterior aspect of the anastomosis between the pancreatic duct and the jejunum is being carried out. When completed, the Portex tube is sutured in place.

75 The outer anterior layer of the pancreaticojejunal anastomosis is next completed.

75

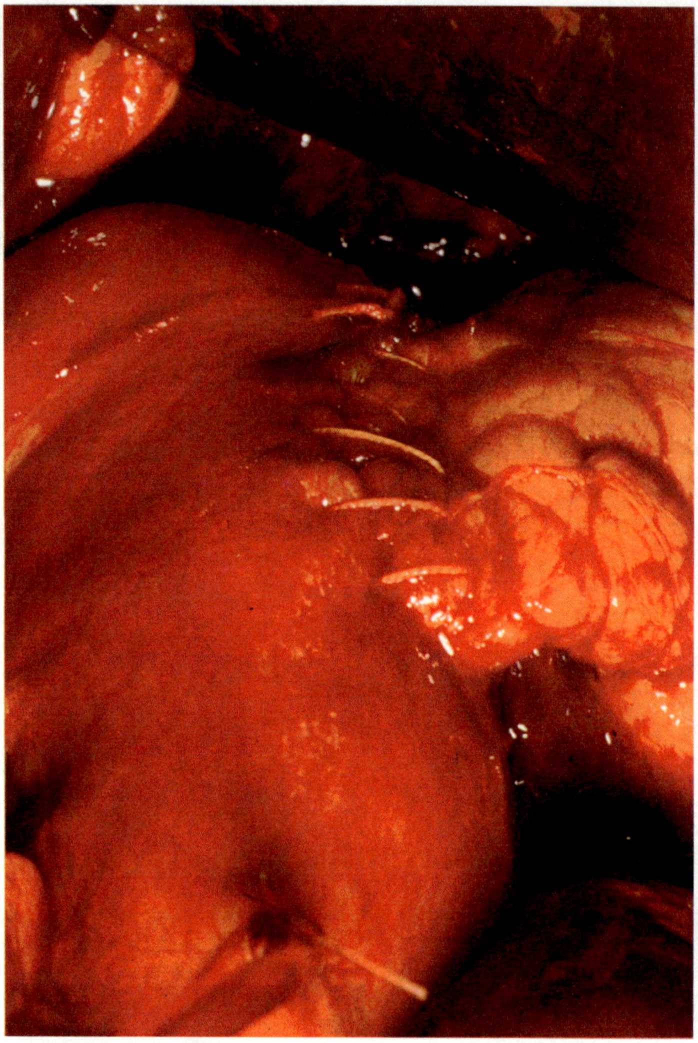

76

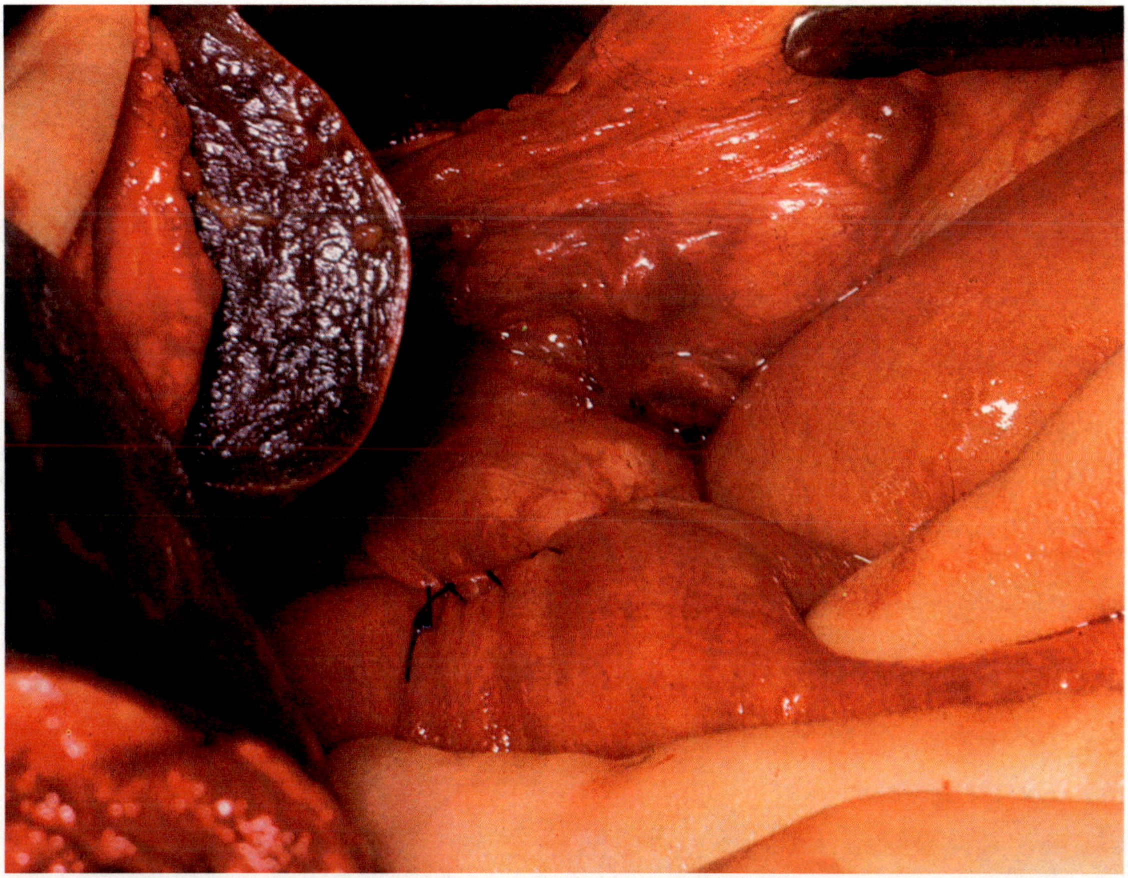

76 **The completed anastomosis in the second case is shown here.**

77

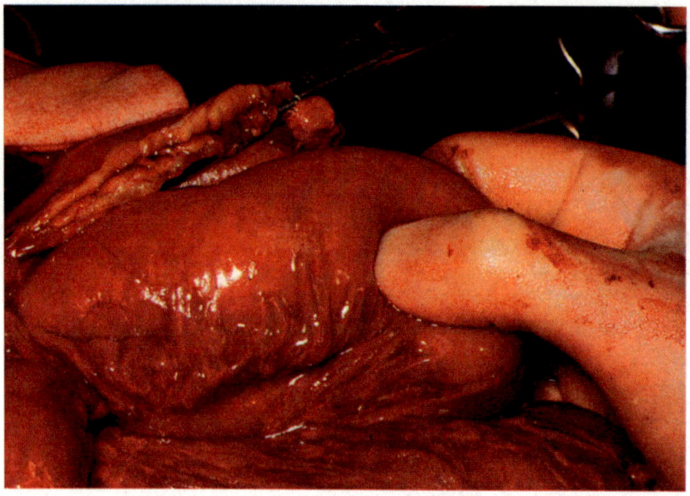

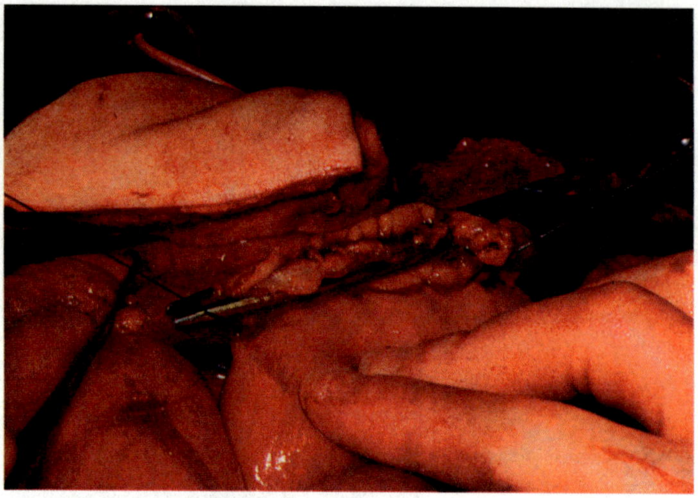

77 and 78 The posterior seromuscular layer of the gastric anastomosis is here being carried out with continuous suture material. A loop of jejunum, about 8 cm distal to the pancreatic anastomosis, is used and an end-to-side gastrojejunal anastomosis is performed.

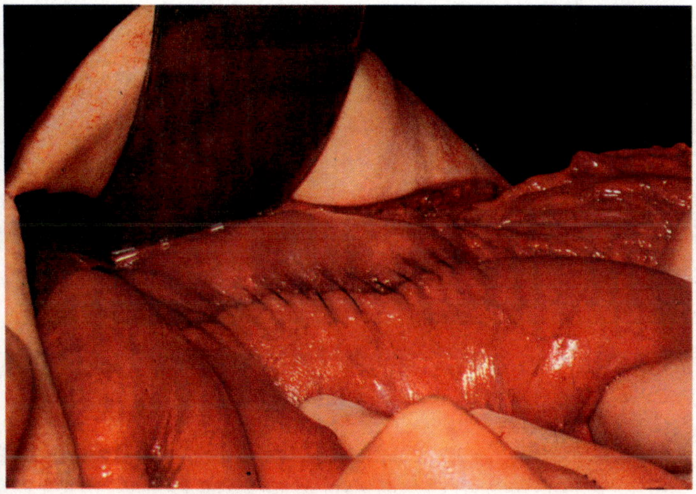

79 The completed two-layer gastrojejunal anastomosis is shown here.

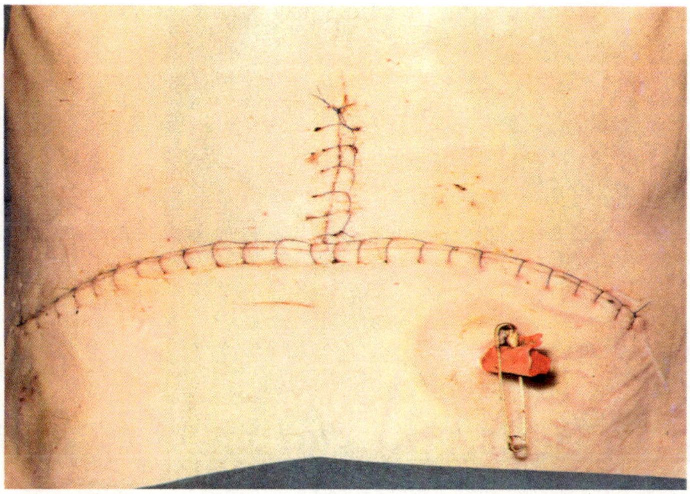 80

80 The abdomen is closed in layers; a drain is inserted into the peritoneal cavity.

81

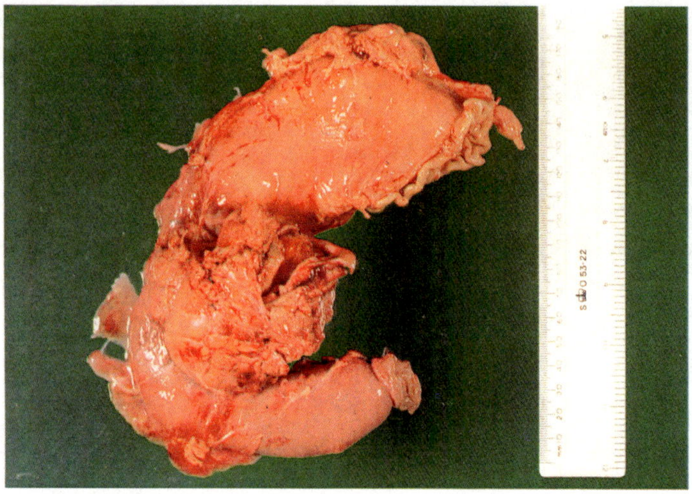

81 **Resected specimen of early pancreatic tumour.**

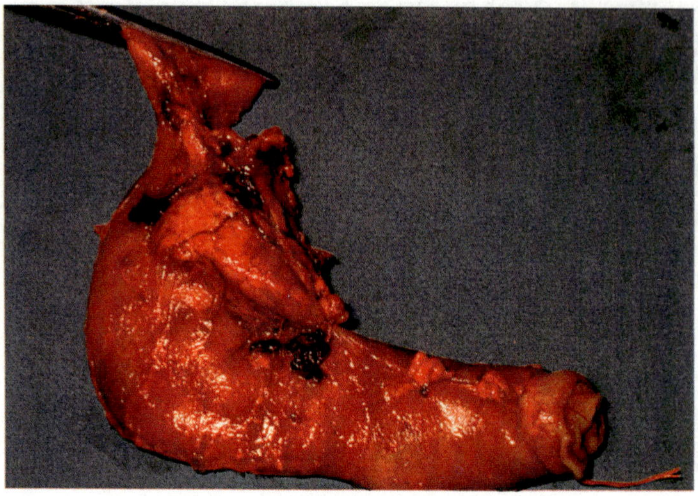

82 **Resected specimen of bile duct tumour.**

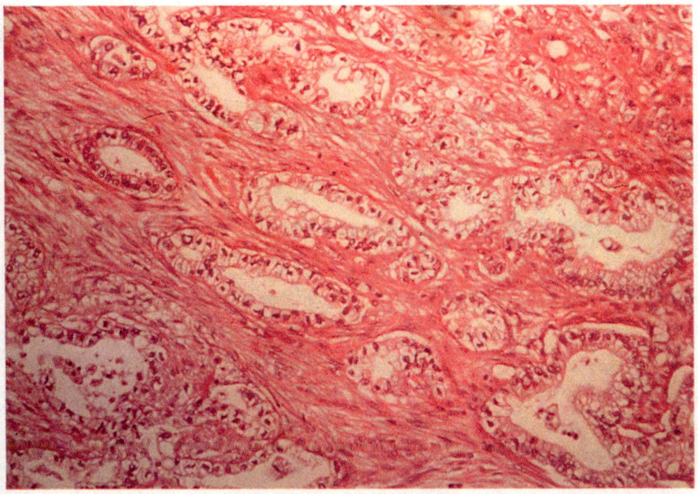

84

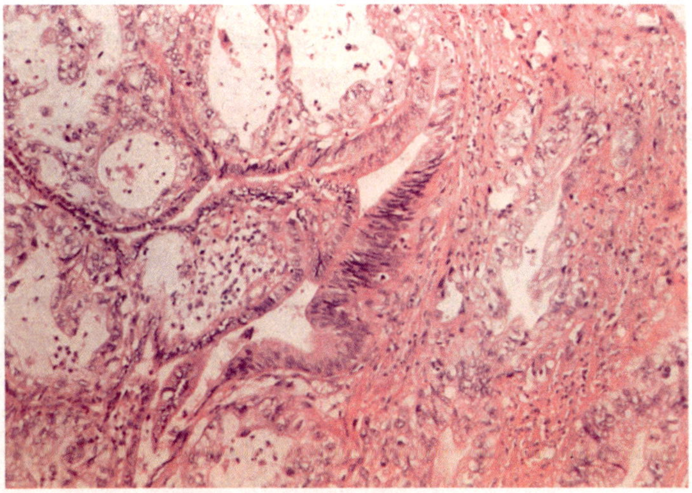

83 Histological specimen of the tumour – a typical bile duct tumour.

84 Histological specimen of the pancreatic tumour.

Transduodenal excision of an ampullary carcinoma

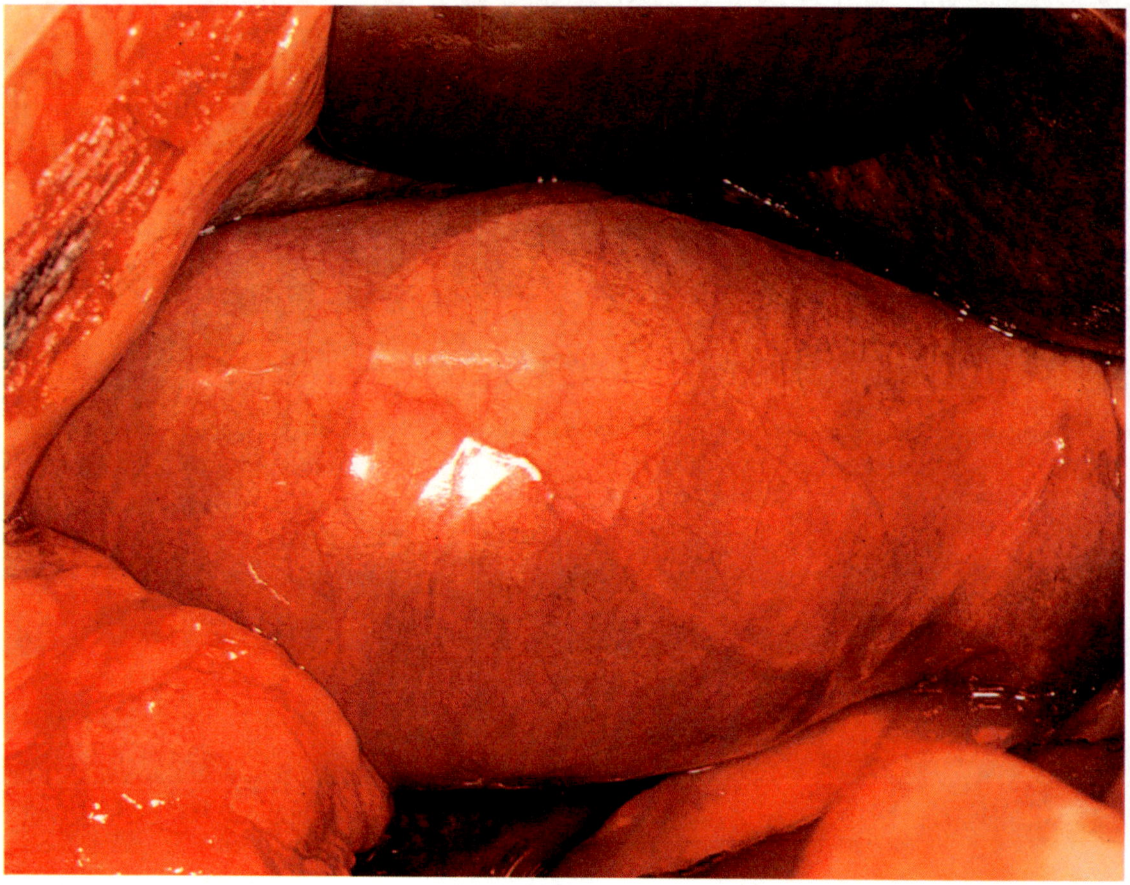

85 Carcinoma of ampulla of Vater. In this patient, 84 years of age, a carcinoma of the ampulla of Vater had caused complete obstruction of the biliary tree. Again, in accordance with Courvoisier's law, gross dilatation of the gallbladder is present.

86

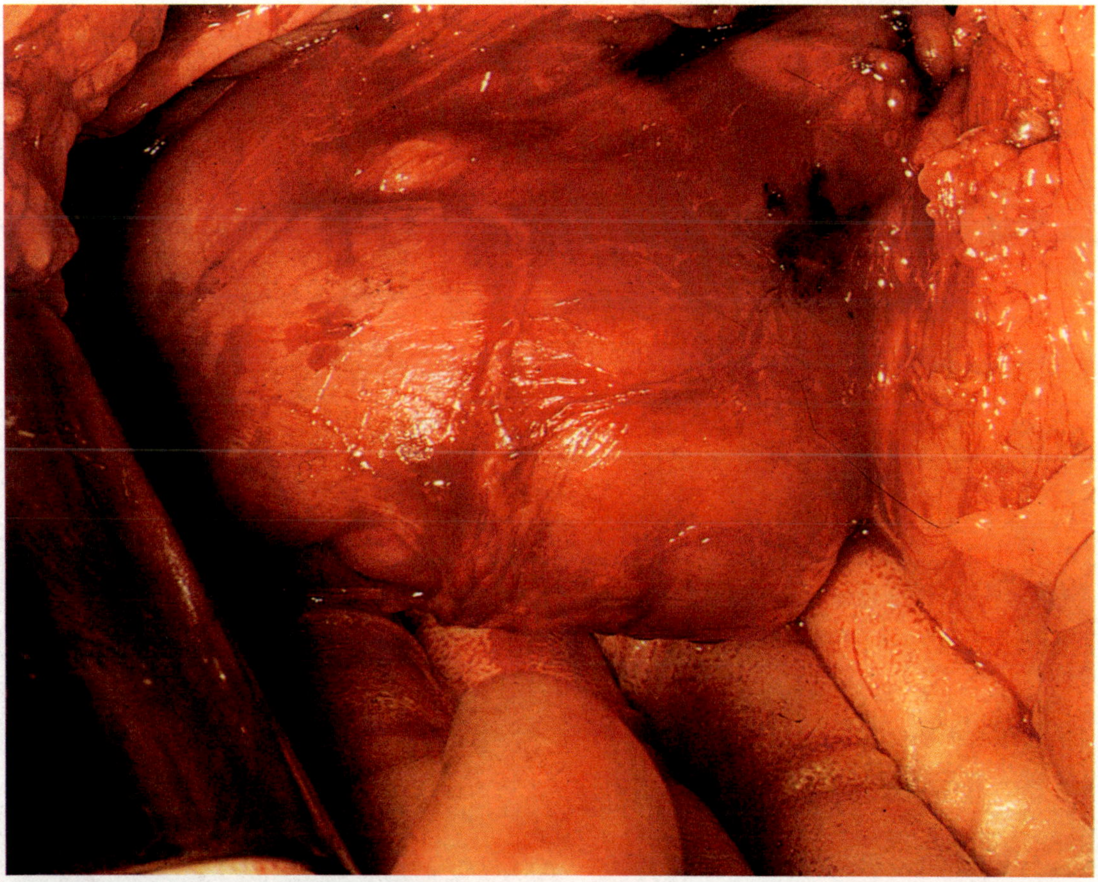

86 The duodenum is mobilised and lifted clear of the posterior abdominal wall.

87

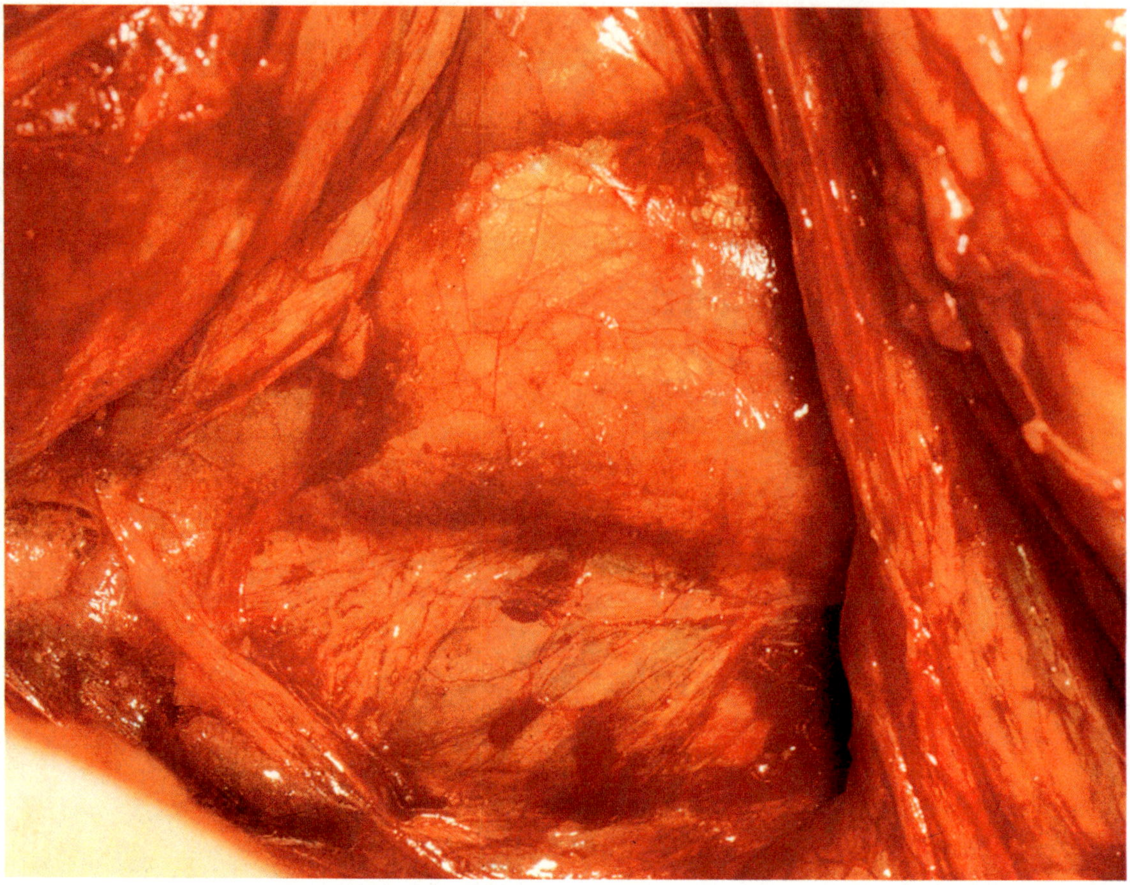

87 The duodenal loop is lifted clear of the inferior vena cava.

88

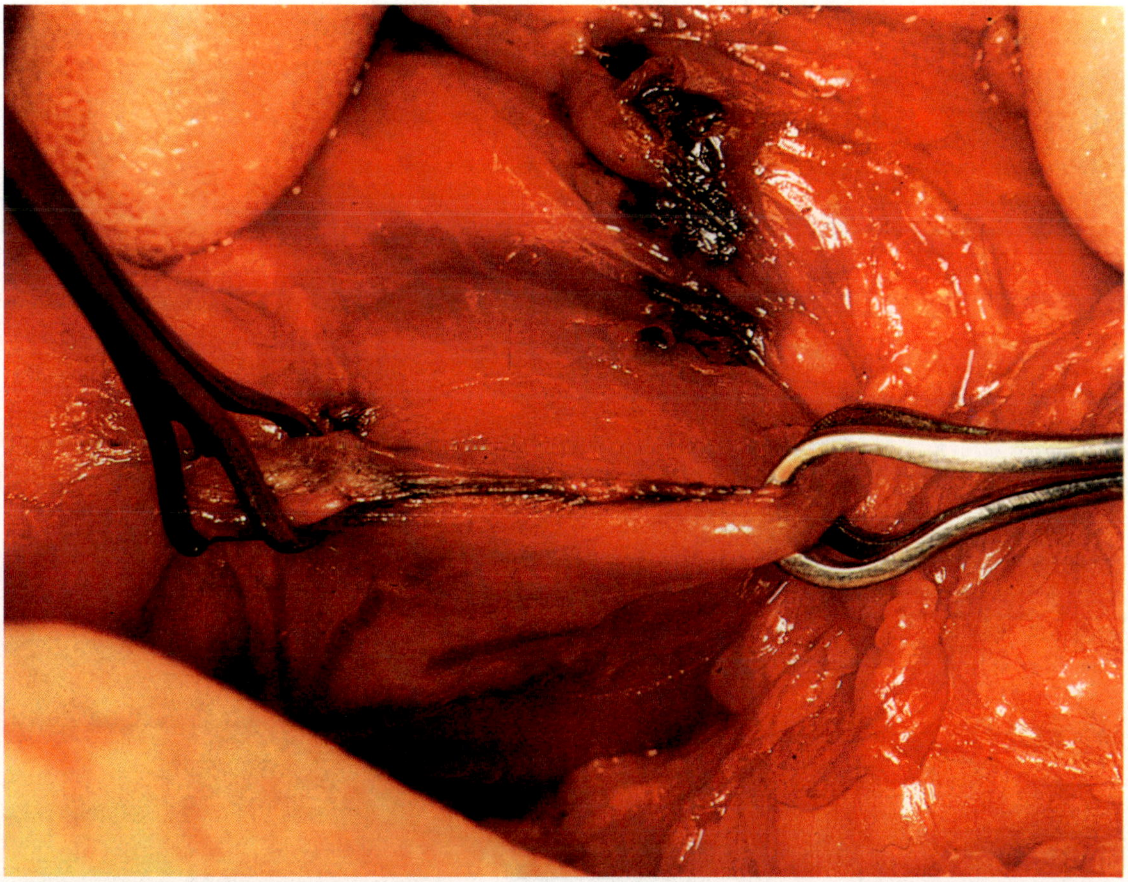

88 The lateral aspect of the second part of the duodenum, opposite the ampullary tumour, is held between Babcock's forceps.

89

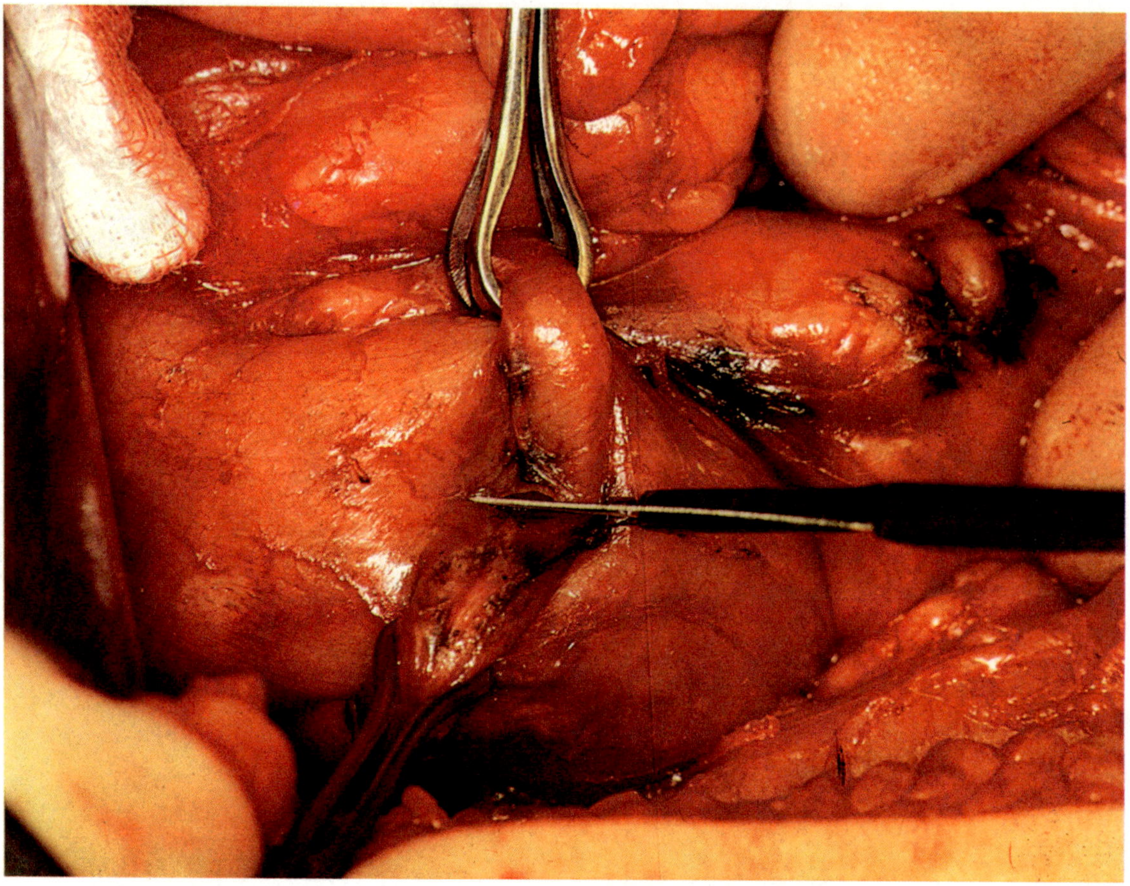

89 A longitudinal incision is made in the duodenum, between the forceps.

90

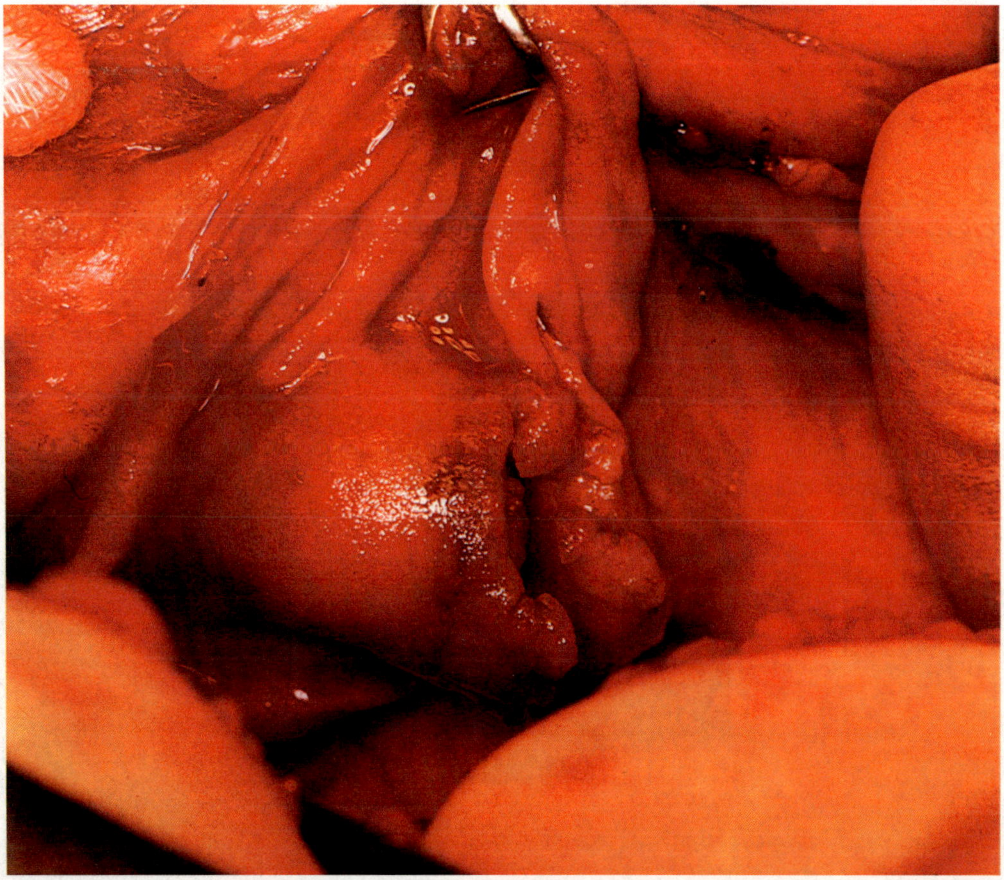

90 The duodenum is opened to reveal the presence of an ulcerated ampullary tumour; this is prolapsed through the duodenotomy.

91 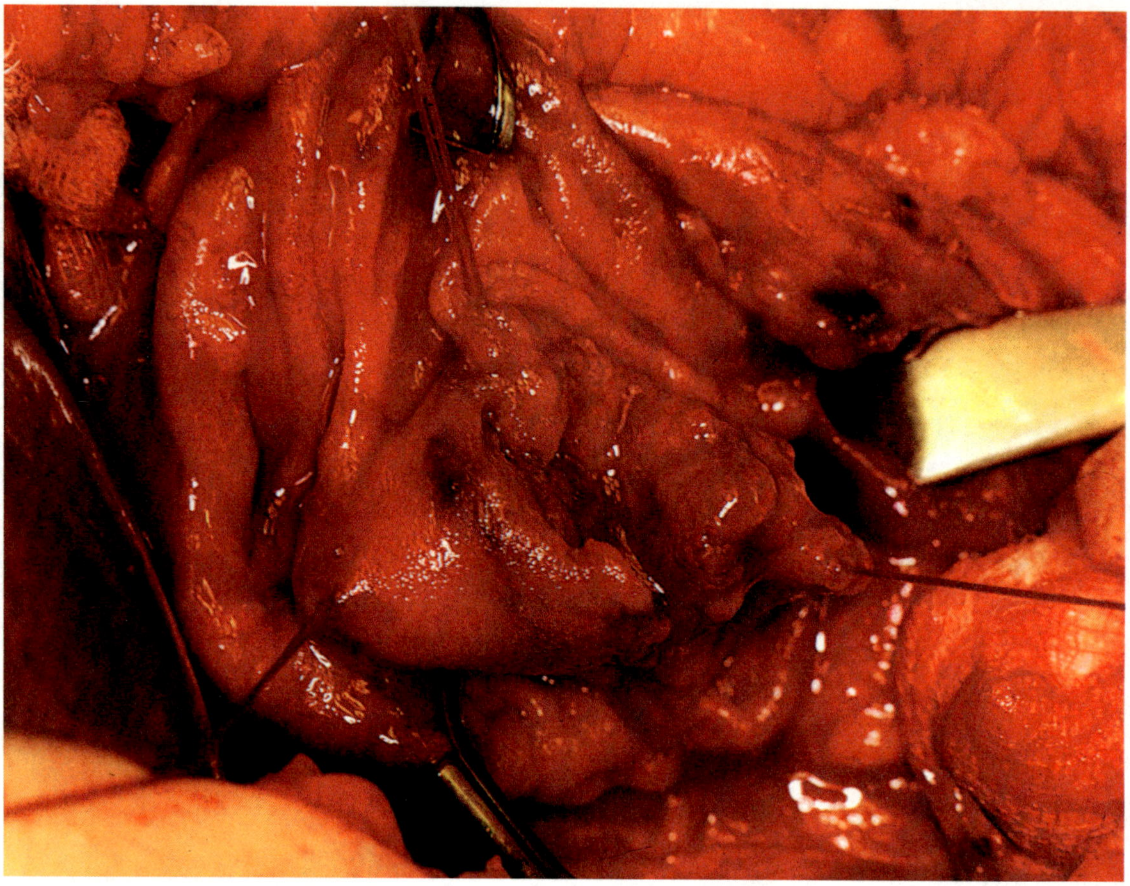

91 Stay-sutures are applied to normal duodenal mucosa, adjacent to the base of the tumour.

92

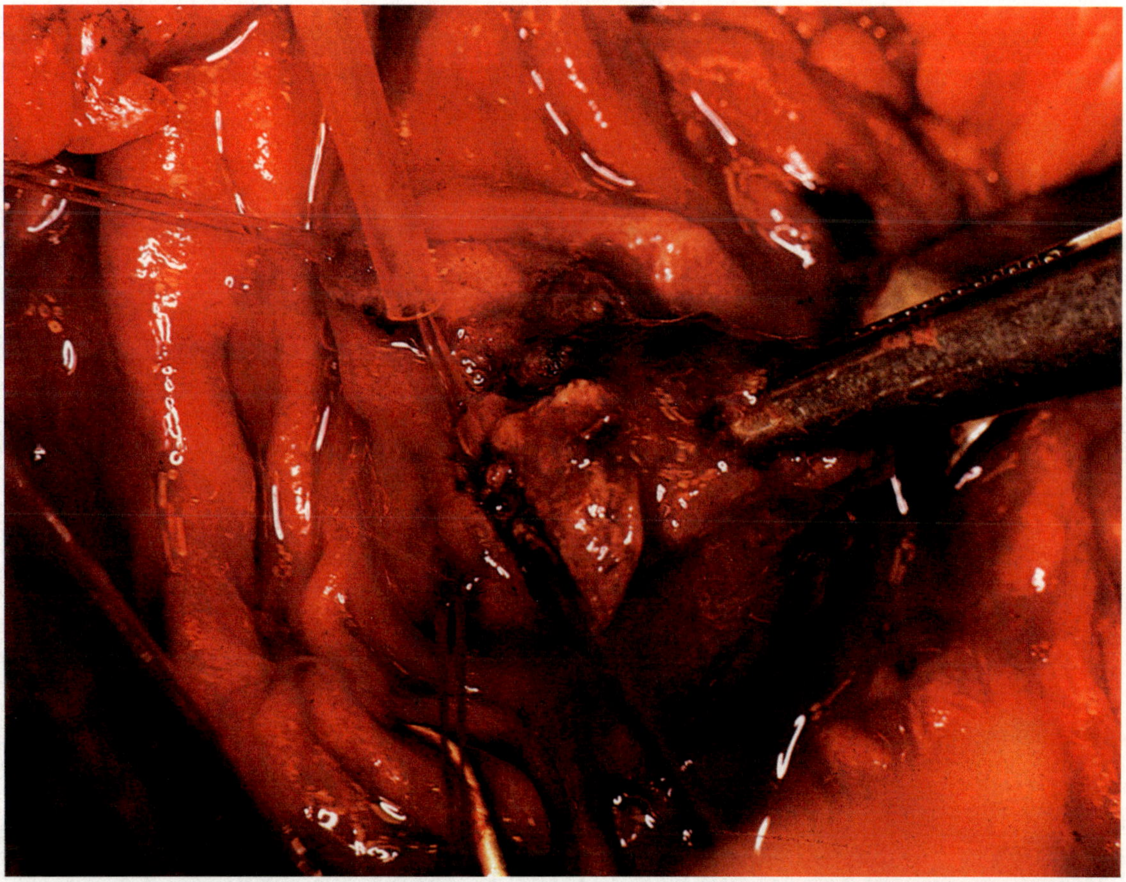

92 **Using a needle diathermy, the duodenal mucosa is incised circumferentially, and the tumour is circumcised.**

93

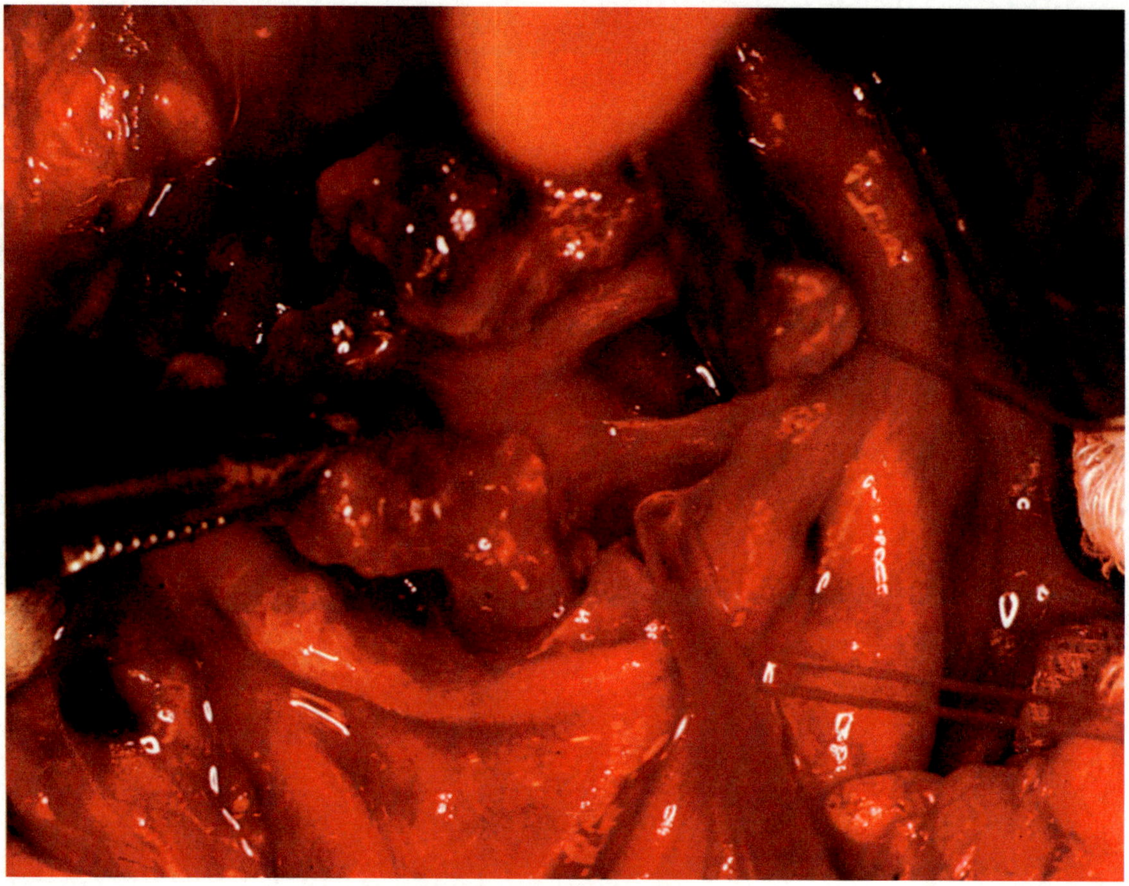

93 The tumour has here been almost completely mobilised, but remains attached inferiorly. The grossly dilated common channel between the bile and pancreatic ducts is identified by the pair of forceps on the right. The forceps on the left retract the tumour away from the underlying ducts.

94

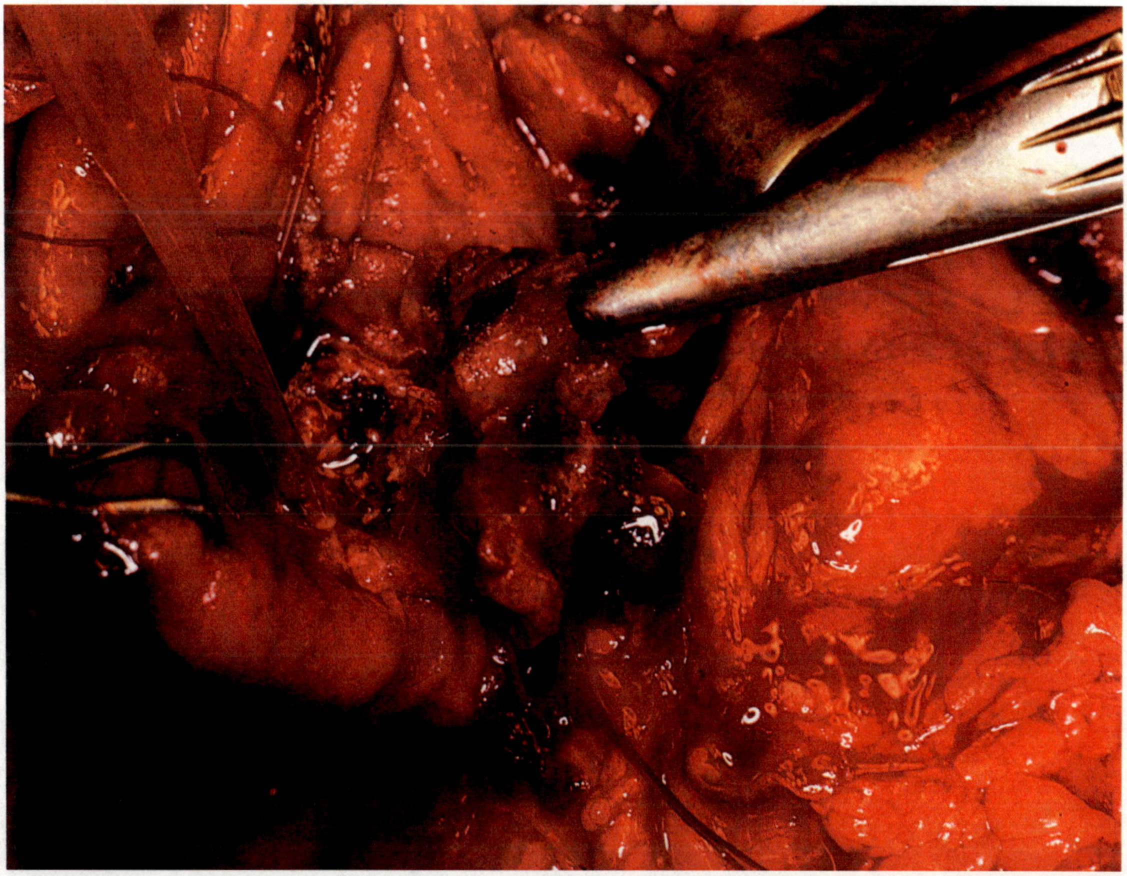

94 The base of the tumour is now excised. Pancreatic tissue can be seen through the duodenal defect. A series of stay-sutures are placed around the edge of the defect to facilitate subsequent closure.

95

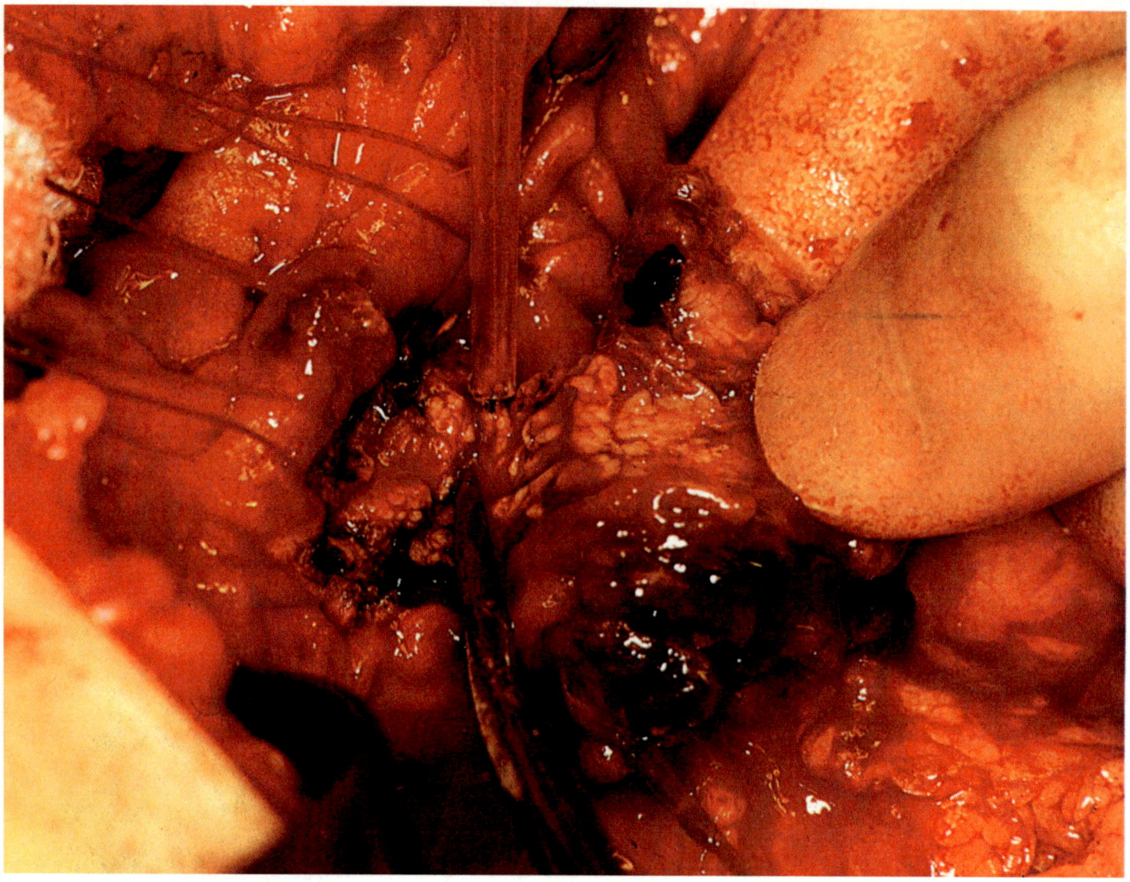

95 The final dissection of the tumour is now taking place.

96

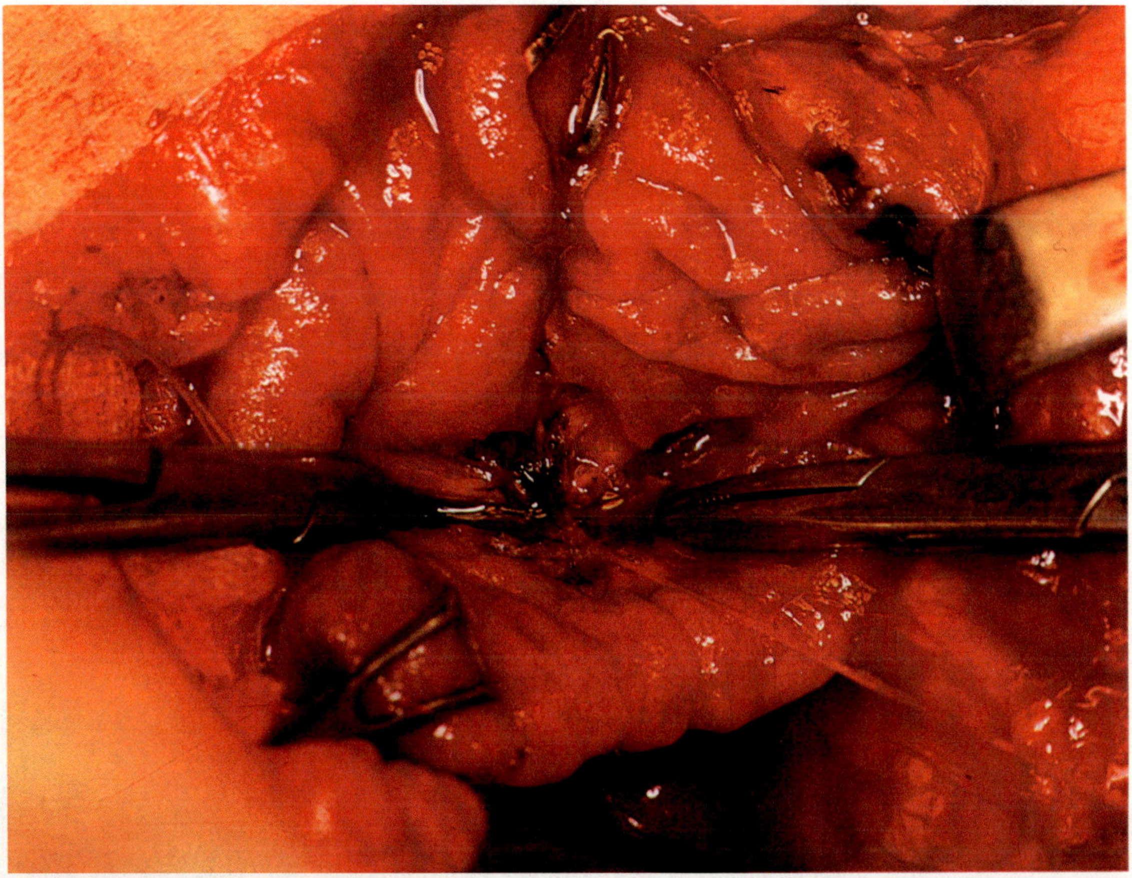

96 The duodenum is now anastomosed around the dilated duct; the duodenal defect is closed in this way.

97

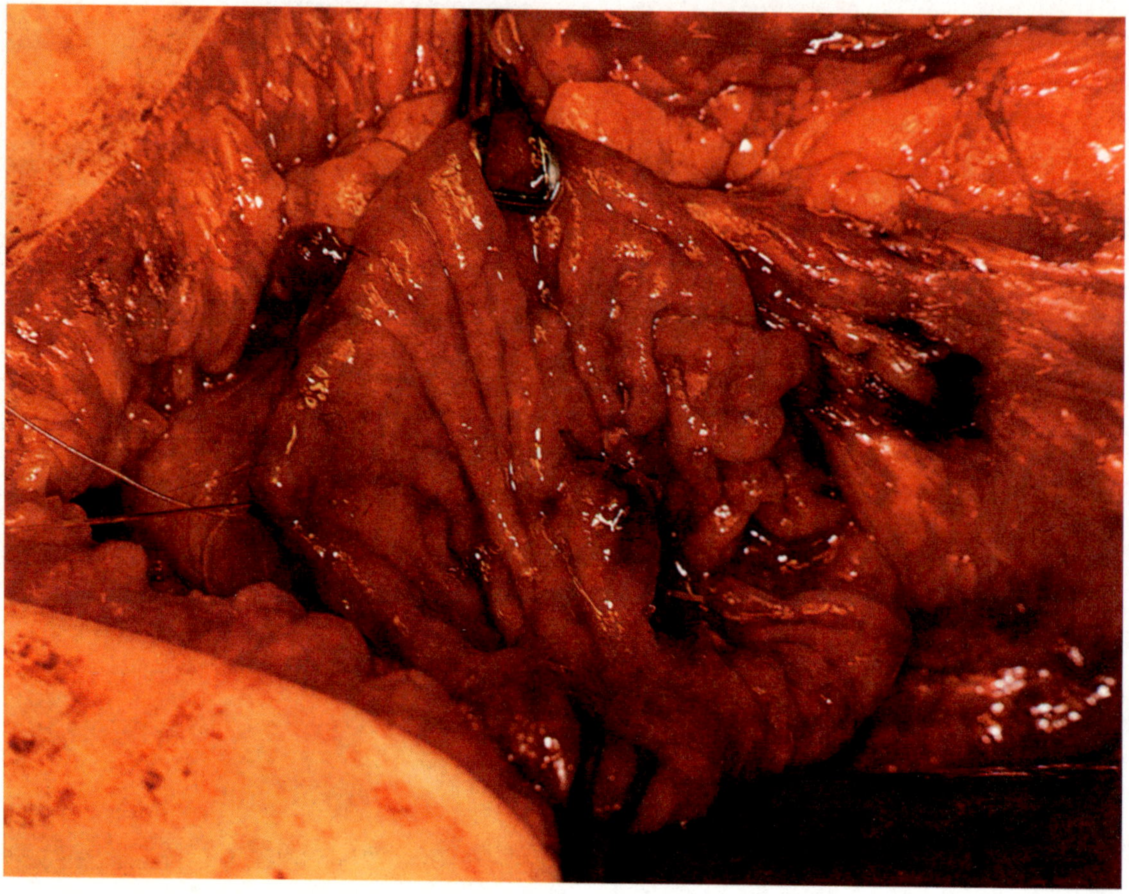

97 The duodenal defect has here been closed around the termination of the bile and pancreatic ducts.

98

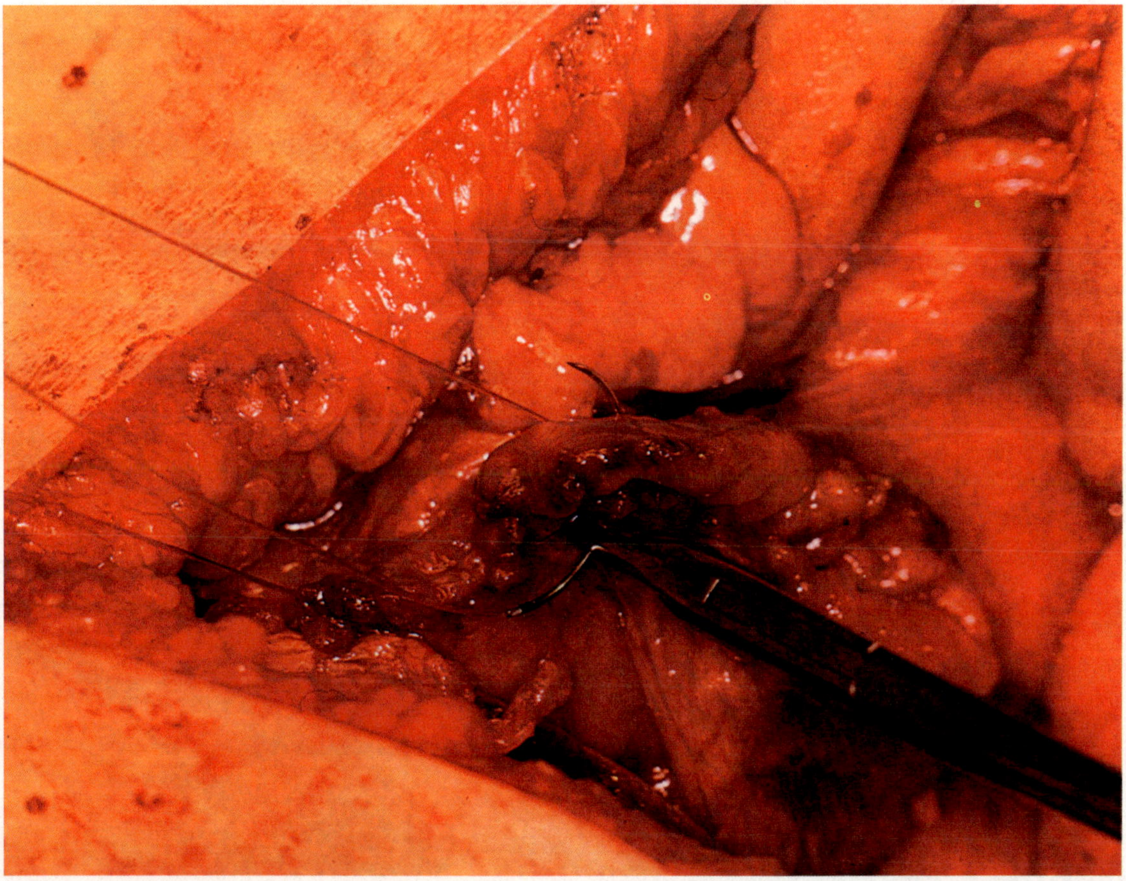

98 The duodenotomy is closed with catgut.

99

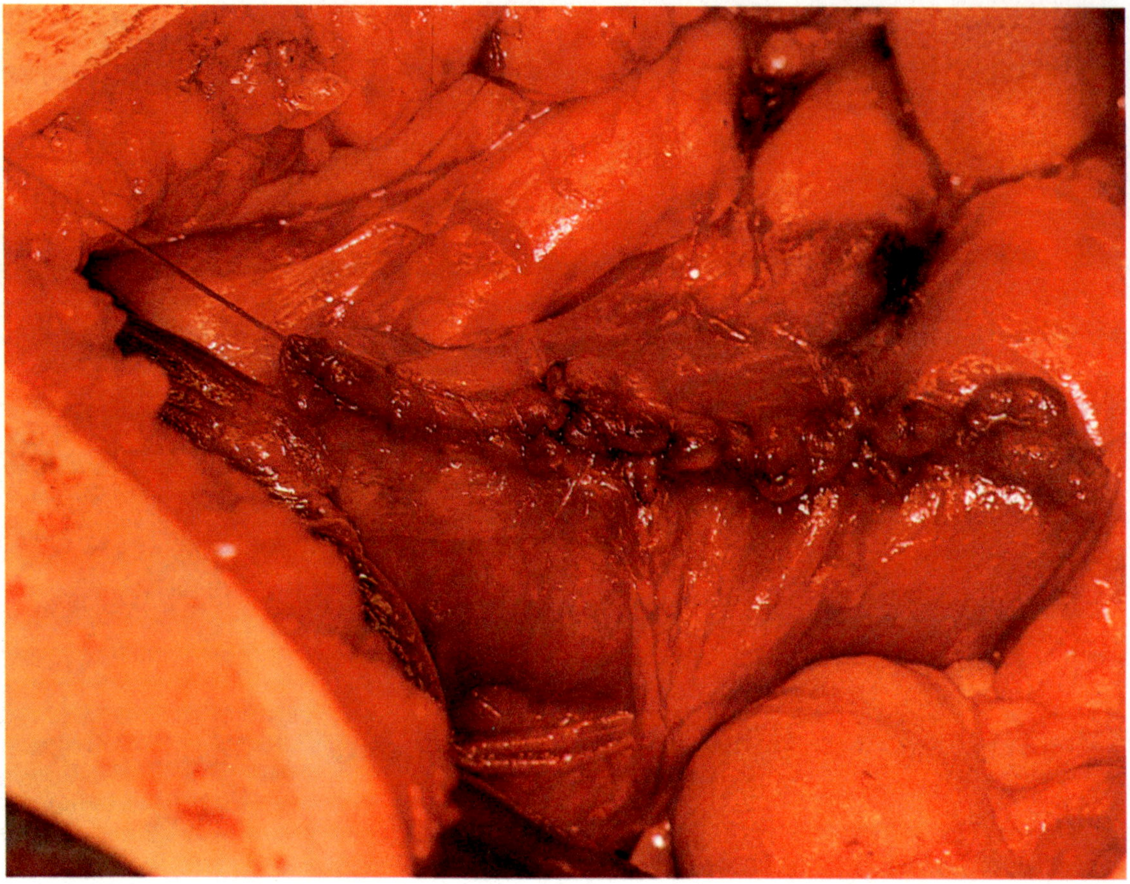

99 The full thickness, deep layer of sutures has completely closed the duodenotomy.

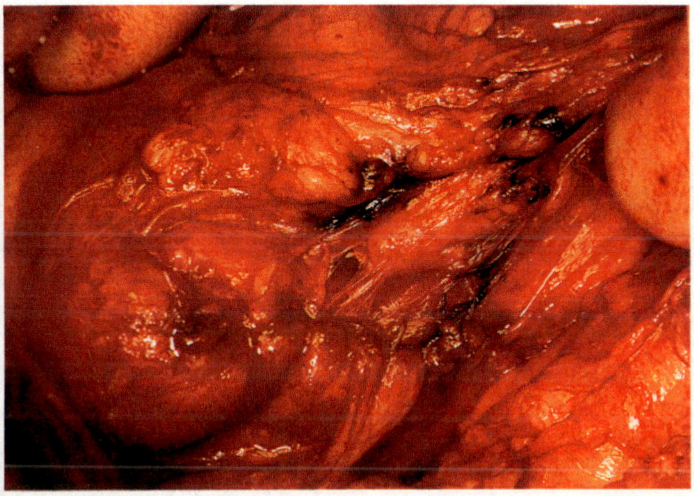

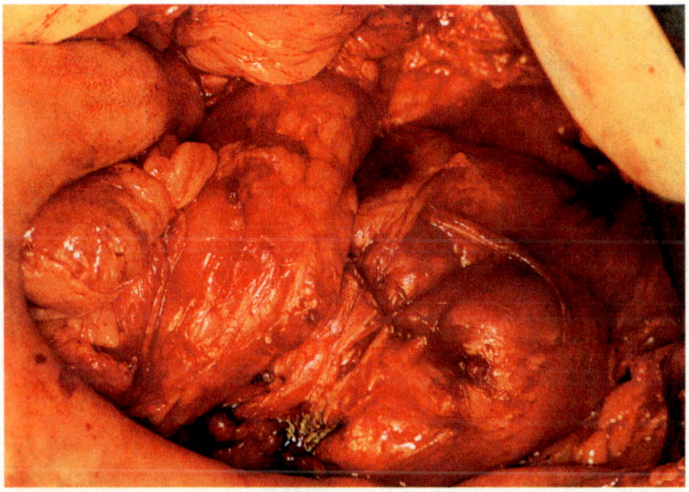

101

100 and 101 A superficial seromuscular layer is inserted to reinforce the deeper layer and to complete the closure.

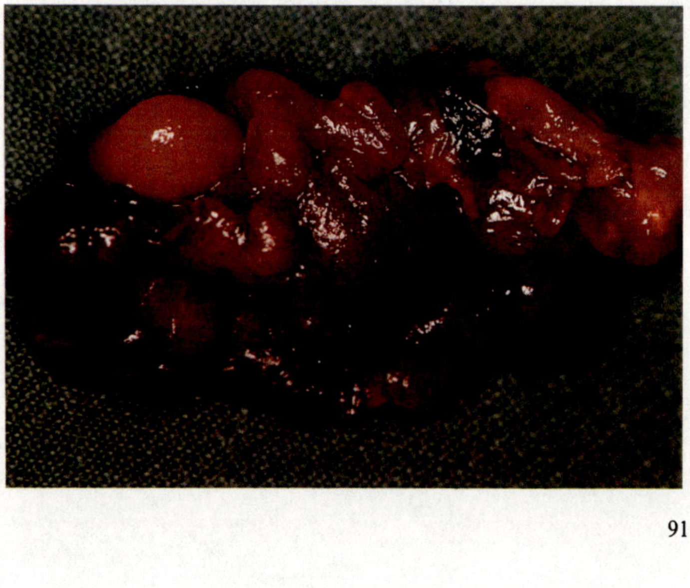

102

102 The excised ampullary tumour.

103

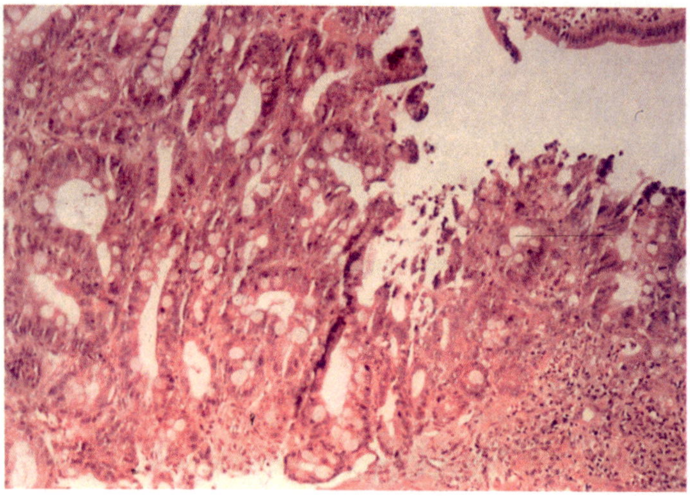

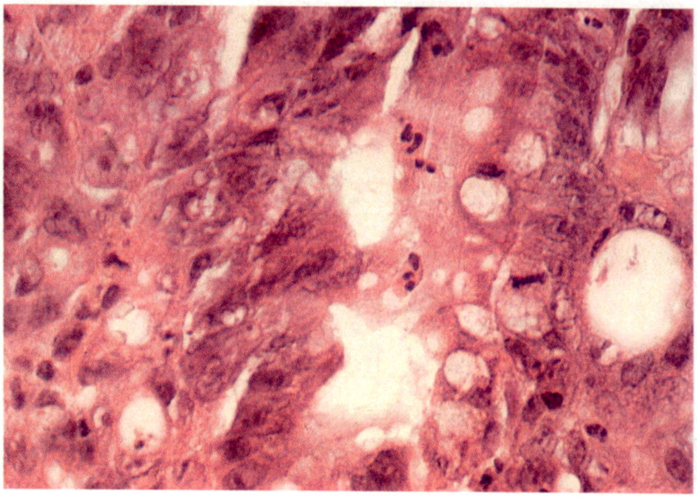

1

103 and 104 Histological sections of the carcinoma of the ampulla of Vater. (Low power × 40, High power × 170.)

Carcinoma of the body of the pancreas

This condition carries an extremely poor prognosis. By the time the condition has manifested itself clinically, it has usually spread by direct invasion into adjacent structures. Resection is rarely possible but if so, should take the form of distal or total pancreatectomy. There are no five-year survivors for carcinoma of the body of the pancreas reported in world medical literature.

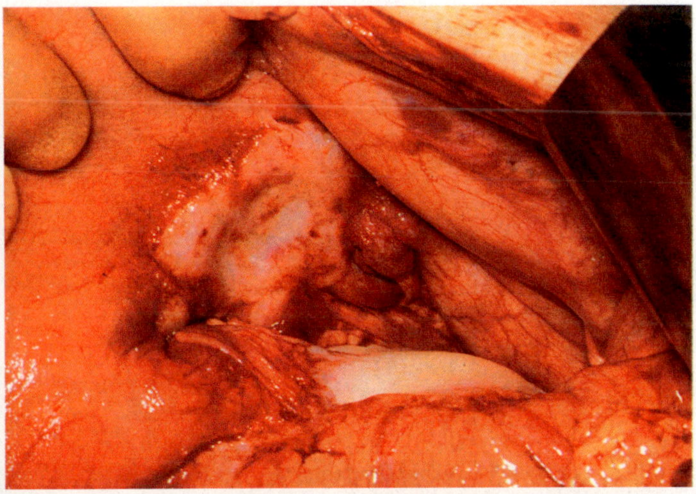

105 Carcinoma of pancreas. The white plaque in the centre of the field is a carcinoma of the body of the pancreas, which has directly invaded the posterior wall of the body of the stomach, giving rise to the large white plaque of tumour seen in the upper left of the field.

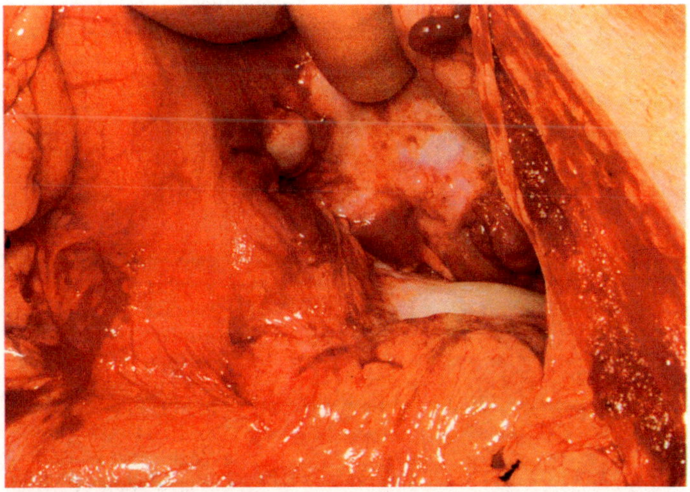

106 Localised portal hypertension has been produced by this tumour, as can be seen from the grossly dilated splenic vein which lies beyond the tumour and behind the gastric deposit. This tumour was fixed and unresectable.

Index

All numbers refer to page numbers only.

MIX
Papier | Fördert gute Waldnutzung
FSC® C083411

Zeitfracht Medien GmbH
Ferdinand-Jühlke-Straße 7
99095 Erfurt, Deutschland
produktsicherheit@kolibri360.de